BALANCED BABES

Every Woman's Guide to Hormone Harmony

STACEY A FOAT

First published by Ultimate World Publishing 2019
Copyright © 2019 Stacey A Foat

ISBN

Paperback - 978-1-925884-57-9
Ebook - 978-1-925884-58-6

Stacey A Foat has asserted her right under the Copyright, Designs and Patents Act 1988 to be identified as the author of this work. The information in this book is based on the author's experiences and opinions. The publisher specifically disclaims responsibility for any adverse consequences, which may result from use of the information contained herein. Permission to use information has been sought by the author. Any breaches will be rectified in further editions of the book.

All rights reserved. No part of this publication may be reproduced, stored in or introduced into a retrieval system, or transmitted in any form, or by any means (electronic, mechanical, photocopying, recording or otherwise) without the prior written permission of the author. Any person who does any unauthorised act in relation to this publication may be liable to criminal prosecution and civil claims for damages. Enquiries should be made through the publisher.

Cover design: Ultimate World Publishing
Layout and typesetting: Ultimate World Publishing
Editor: Hayley Ward

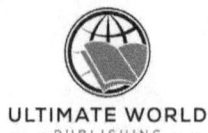

Ultimate World Publishing
Diamond Creek,
Victoria Australia 3089
www.writeabook.com.au

To my beautiful Dad, my painful reminder that mainstream medicine alone doesn't always have the answers. RIP Gregory Charles Foat xx

CONTENTS

Introduction vii

PART 1: 'THE ART OF BALANCE' 1
Chapter 1: Girl, it ain't your hormones 3
Chapter 2: Be a SELFish bitch 17
Chapter 3: O DEAR 25
Chapter 4: The problem with the pill 37

PART 2: 'THE 7 STEP HORMONE HEALING SYSTEM' 51
Chapter 5: Girl, you're a HOT mess 57
Chapter 6: Releasing your shit 75
Chapter 7: What's bugging you? 89
Chapter 8: This girl is on fire 109
Chapter 9: Your gut is your guru 121
Chapter 10: Nailing Nutrition 139
Chapter 11: Emotional evolution 157
Chapter 12: Balanced & beautiful 171

Afterword 187
About The Author 189
Acknowledgements 193

INTRODUCTION

I remember the exact look on my endocrinologist's face when she exclaimed I had, "more than likely" commenced menopause. I imagine the look of horror on my face was what prompted her to cheerfully add, as if it was no big deal, "don't worry, IVF has come a long way, you can freeze embryos and I'm sure you'll still be able to have a family". As if that was some kind of consolation prize that a single, 27-year-old woman who in that moment was feeling like a complete failure needed to hear.

It all started when I decided to 'quit sugar'. Worst idea ever! I should have known better than to deprive myself of my one great love - chocolate. After years of, as my mother would put it, "burning the candle at both ends," late night partying, working full-time, studying and socialising as if my life depended on it, I officially burnt myself out.

The truth is, I had always had 'issues' concerning my period but as a teenager who felt embarrassed about even getting a period, it wasn't exactly lunchtime conversation with my friends or family so how was I to know my periods weren't normal? I generally bled every 17-21 days and it was super heavy. I had resigned to the fact that I had to line my bed with old towels each time I had my period, and since I could manage the level of pain with Nurofen it wasn't so bad. At high school I lost count of the number of times I had to wear my jumper around my waist because I'd 'leaked' through my clothes and when

I plucked up the courage to learn how to use a tampon years later, I might as well have shoved two supers up there, because they didn't do much when the floods started every few weeks.

This is how things continued through my teenage years and 20's. Then my symptoms really ramped up and my periods became irregular with unexplained weight gain, emotional lows, severe fatigue, hot flushes, pain and bleeding with intercourse and cystic lumpy skin breakouts. It felt like doctors didn't really know what was wrong with me - maybe it was even in my head - but I kept going back hassling for an answer, so this diagnosis will do. Under the mainstream medical model, I was just one of the 'unlucky ones' and the only advice I was given was to try and start conceiving as soon as possible.

As deflated as I was, I wasn't ready to call it quits and I certainly wasn't ready to accept menopause at such a young age, so I dug deep, drew on my naturopathy knowledge and virtually locked myself indoors for the next six months. Having recently relocated to Geelong in winter and not having a social life helped. I didn't even get out of bed most weekends; I just read and researched everything and anything about hormones and what the hell mine were up to! Thankfully it didn't take long for me to work out what was going on. Now I needed to find out why it was happening and not merely mask it with the 'Pill' as the GP and endocrinologist had recommended.

Adrenal exhaustion - that's pretty much what was going on in my body causing my symptoms.

So, let's go back to the start, the fun part that got me in this mess in the beginning. In my early twenties, I was living large, partying lots and having an awesome time. I had a huge tribe of outgoing girlfriends. We danced, partied and socialised at least four nights a week. At least two, sometimes three of these days involved alcohol - large amounts of alcohol. Because I was studying a Nutrition and Naturopathy degree, I had enough knowledge to look after myself pretty well. I ate great, exercised lots and knew a bit about self-care. I rarely got hangovers and never got sick, which pretty much just meant I could push the limits

INTRODUCTION

even further. I'd always been a bit of a sugar junkie, so to compensate I was strict with my exercise. In fact, it wasn't uncommon for me to go for a run on the beach in the morning, then saddle up to a gym session or class in the evening, which was usually with my girlfriends so we could go out and drink calories in the form of alcohol or eat ice cream straight after! To us, that was balance!

Fast forward the clock five years, there'd been lots of late nights (or should I say early mornings), and lots of abusing my body in general. The cracks were beginning to show. Emotionally I was low, and all of a sudden, I didn't enjoy the party scene anymore. I was single, lonely and depressed. I knew it was time for a change; time to start looking after myself and focusing on self-care. So, I did what everyone else was doing at the time and put myself on a Paleo diet, quitting sugar and carbs. I was sure this would help me to feel better and kick the couple of kg's that had crept on over the years. But this was actually the worst thing I could have done. Because my adrenal glands were so frazzled from lack of sleep, over-training, overuse of stimulants (alcohol and sugar) and 'burning the candle at both ends,' when I deprived them of that quick hit of energy, they basically went into meltdown. My adrenals were officially fatigued.

Think of hormones like dominoes - if one is out of whack, eventually the whole pack are disrupted. That's what was going on with me. My thyroid slowed down due to shortages of thyroid hormones from the inflammation and stress in my body. My body couldn't balance the oestrogen and progesterone, so my periods became super irregular, and with the sudden cessation of sugar and alcohol, my body went into detox mode, which is kind of good, but in this case, it was kind of bad because I was too depleted and adrenally stressed for my body to do a good job of it. So, I was releasing toxins in all the wrong places, which caused acne, headaches, mood swings, digestive problems, weight gain and fatigue. On top of this, because my liver was so sluggish from all the partying and high sugar, I had candida overgrowth, eczema and had developed elevated kryptopyrrole molecules in my body which literally made me feel CRAZY! Anxiety, paranoia, depression, irritability and all the associated mood swings. Mentally and physically, I was a mess. It was the lowest period of my life, and I'm just so thankful my university degree enabled me to make sense of exactly what was going on, otherwise I'd probably still be suffering, five years on, like many women are.

This story does have a happy ending, though. It only took me a solid six months to clean up the mess, but it had to be done correctly, in a specific order. I couldn't restore my thyroid health until my adrenals were up and running. I couldn't nourish my adrenal glands until I healed my digestion and corrected my diet. I couldn't lose weight until I stimulated my liver. I couldn't manage my moods until I corrected the nutritional deficiencies. I couldn't reduce the inflammation before detoxing the chemicals. I couldn't detox before restoring the adrenals. And I was never going to restore my adrenals until the candida infection was eradicated.

Although it seemed complex, through understanding how the body intricately worked and related to each system I was able to reverse all the debilitating symptoms with simple lifestyle changes and nutritional and herbal medicine, based on healing and treating the body at a cellular level by addressing the cause of the dysfunctional hormones. I shudder to think how very different the outcome could have been if it wasn't for my knowledge in the natural medicine field.

So, if like me you're experiencing hormone hell, or you are committed to preventing chronic disease, this book is for you! In fact, this book is for anyone who has an interest in self-care, feeling and looking your best and taking personal responsibility for your health. Holistic health isn't always the quickest and easiest option but it's the safest, most sustainable approach in the long run, and your body will love you for it!

PART 1

'THE ART OF BALANCE'

CHAPTER 1

GIRL, IT AIN'T YOUR HORMONES

"Nothing changes if nothing changes."
Annonymous

It's time I hit you with some hard truths. I figure we'll get it over and done with straight up, like a band-aid; rip it off quickly and be done with it. It may shock you a little, but it's the best way to get to the bottom of all these modern-day misconceptions and ultimately save you from years of 'hormone hell'.

So, here's the thing. Your hormones aren't to blame for anything. Now before you get pissed off that maybe you bought the wrong bloody book, because you have the blood test results, urinary tests or even saliva samples which 'prove' your hormones are out of balance, or everything you've read on the internet indicates you have a hormonal imbalance… I want you to understand this one thing. Your hormones are simply the messengers. They are produced, stimulated, and sent all over the body to hormone receptor sites in response to physiological changes which occur within your body. Physiological changes which are brought about by anything and everything that has an influence on the functioning of your body.

It's a nifty little process called homeostasis, and it keeps everything in check in your body despite the ever-changing environment we live in. So, when the temperature outside changes or your body becomes massively acidic after that double shot espresso, or when your heart rate increases because your partner is pissing you off or you've skipped a meal and your blood sugar levels start to plummet, and all the thousands of other things which occur daily, your body still has to maintain balance. We can't afford for our body to lose its shit or go on holidays; everything in your body has a specific working range, like your blood pH, your heart rate, your breathing rate, your kidneys filtration rate and so on. All these amazing biological processes which keep us alive occur due to thousands of cellular processes occurring every single second. And our cells use hormones to signal these physiological changes which need to occur in the body to bring about rapid change when shit starts to go down, also known as something is out of whack in your body threatening your health.

Our environment is changing every single minute, but your body needs to stay within strict boundaries to ensure optimal health (that's how your insides don't cook when you are in the sauna). The problem is, there's a whole heap of things that affect the 'balance' of our body; the foods we eat, the liquids we consume, the lack of water we consume, the toxins we're exposed to, our thoughts and emotions, medications, stressful situations, our energy consumption, how much sleep we're getting and so on. All of these things affect our body, which means they affect what hormones are produced, when they are produced and how much of them! So, you see it's not the fault of your hormones; they are merely responding to the changes that are occurring in your body in every moment. Actually, come to think of it, your hormones are actually life savers.

Which leads me to truth bomb number 2….it's not your doctor's, your specialist's, your gyno's, or even your naturopath's job to 'heal' you. Only you can do that, by first recognising where you went wrong in the first place.

Disease is never random or 'bad luck'. Disease is ALWAYS the consequence of your physical environment, emotional state and spiritual health. That is what we call holistic health; encompassing all elements of health and not merely compartmentalising the most sophisticated creation on the planet as though it were a Lego man. PS, I'm talking about humans. When we take ownership, it's like jumping in the driver's seat and taking back control. This allows us to start making choices that support our health, listening to the body and taking actions which support our longevity and ability to feel frickin' awesome. Body, mind and soul.

The emerging awareness surrounding debilitating conditions, painful fricken things like endometriosis, polycystic ovarian syndrome and hypothyroidism leading to infertility, acne, weight gain, low self-esteem and depression is a positive step in the right direction. But without offering any practical tools to reverse and heal these conditions, merely feeding women bullshit about these conditions being 'incurable' only leaves women feeling more powerless than before.

We can't let these horrid conditions win, and that's what we're doing when we keep giving away our power, expecting someone else to ease our pain or take the 'quick fix' approach like pharmaceuticals, surgery and even more drastic approaches like hysterectomies and mastectomies.

Don't get me wrong, all of these medical procedures have a place, but if you're not willing to listen to your body and find out why it developed this disease or imbalance in the first place then what's the point; the disease is only going to manifest somewhere else in the body.

If you're only willing to suppress your body's cry for help with drugs or surgery, you'll be stuck in your diagnosis forever which is only going to lead you down a dangerous path of hormone hell with much more serious consequences in the future. Look at the leading causes of death among women worldwide – breast cancer and heart disease, neither of which occur overnight or completely due to bad luck. Both of these conditions were simmering away in the background, and your body was trying to let you know through uncomfortable sensations and feelings of emotional disconnect for many years before they reared themselves 'large' enough for medical equipment to be able to identify and diagnose.

Please believe me babe, I feel you. I've been there. You read the intro, right? This is not about blaming you or making you feel crap about your lifestyle; this is about giving you back the power because when we know better, we can do better. It's about helping you to pull your head out of the misconceptions and fear the media is flooding you with and getting to the truth. This is about equipping you with the education and tools to help you make the positive changes your body is screaming out for. It's about teaching you how to understand your body and gain the confidence to ask the right questions and learn what is right for you, which of course is going to be completely different to old love down the street. And most importantly, it's about balance. Hey, I'm a self-confessed chocoholic, and I love me some chemical hair straightening and a loose night out on the wines with my girlfriends. Being healthy isn't about living in a prison cell of mung beans, a strict yoga regime and NO fun, it's just about recognising what your body needs and giving it to it as much as you possibly can, whilst enjoying every minute of the day….coffee, wine, chocolate and all!

Don't let your diagnosis define you. Better yet, don't let the diagnosis occur at all. Focus your efforts on prevention, which will always be far more powerful than trying to reverse the damage after it's done.

Breast cancer rates continue to soar every year, despite new advances in technology and screening. So, what! What good is screening for breast cancer? It ain't going to stop you developing cancer in the first place. Come on, ladies you can do better than that! You have the power to protect your body from these 'common hormonal' conditions, fibroids, irregular cervical cells, ovarian cysts, hot flushes and so on. Sorry, but

I'm going to call it; early detection will never be as good as not getting cancer in the first place and until women are willing to place their health in their OWN hands and take a proactive approach to living well, through understanding what their bodies need, breast cancer rates will continue to climb. It's your body and your responsibility.

While I'm still on my high horse, let me introduce you to the other 'poor victim' of this new age blood bath of dodging responsibility and playing the blame game. Genetics. The old, 'it's not my fault, my mum and my mum's mum had hideous hormones too, it's in our genes'. Sorry that's a cop-out.

And although I'm coming across as a rather nasty cow again (sorry), I'm not the sort of person who gets my kicks bringing a sister down. The truth is, I'm an empath and seeing women suffer to the extremity that they do breaks my heart, which is why my message is so passionate (abrupt and often lacking tact). There's enough research out there proving that our genes are largely influenced by our environment, that is, whether they choose to express themselves or not is completely up to the way you live your life - diet, exercise, stress, emotional well-being, spiritual connection, toxic exposure. BOOM. Are you beginning to see the pattern? We have more control over our health then we have ever dared to believe and even the things that we can't control as an individual, like air pollution and workplace bullies, we can absolutely take a stand for ourselves and protect ourselves from these evil scenarios.

So, whether you're dealing with those beastly ovarian cysts that keep bursting, annoying acne, the ghastly six months pregnant look every time of the month or the fact sex is either a) the last thing you could give a damn about or b) too painful to actually enjoy let alone get your rocks off, either way, you have the power to heal your body and prevent it re-occurring! Do you want to know why it actually makes very little difference as to what you are experiencing and how your 'hormone imbalance' is playing out? Because to heal the body successfully we need to holistically address the causes of 'disease' and give the body what it needs to heal itself, not merely provide some short-term relief from the symptoms.

Remember, in case you are distracted by my tone, I share this info because I care. Because I know that hiding behind blaming our hormones for all the 'female' crap we have to put up with isn't going to change your circumstance anytime soon. I love you and I don't' want you to end up as yet another breast cancer statistic. Your hormones are behaving badly because you and your lifestyle are messing with them. Sorry. Not sorry.

I don't want women to keep giving away their power to the pharmaceutical industry, expecting a drug to fix the problems it's most likely contributing to in the first place.

Only when we take ownership of our body and start listening to what it's trying to tell us, will we be able to take back our power and heal our bodies.

So, here's the recap.

At the risk of getting all fancy 'sciency' (which you've probably figured out isn't really my style) there are a few things we need to understand about our bodies and life in general, so that we can move forward on this hormone harmony journey together.

1. Your body doesn't hate you

Your vagina isn't trying to punish you and your uterus isn't some rogue foreign entity that has invaded your body to try and make your life a living hell.

Actually, it's quite the opposite - our lady bits are actually a pretty cool internal compass. When we connect our heart with our womb and start to understand how our hormones work, we can actually start to feel more powerful and connected than ever before, not to mention the fact we are literally able to create life and bring another human into the world, thanks to this incredible organ.

2. Genes and genetics is somewhat a load of bullshit

Sure, you can keep blaming your endometriosis or your savage PMS on your great great grandma if you want….or you can start living in the 21st century and understand that epigenetics is now where the party is at. You have the ability to signal genes, downregulate them and upregulate them, and turn them on and off based on how well you are looking after your body. Diet, stress levels, toxicity, infection control, thoughts and beliefs matter. Don't believe me? Check out Dr Bruce Lipton's work and his book, The Biology of Belief.

3. Hormones are messengers

They don't actually have a mind of their own and they're not all inside you conspiring against you, trying to kill you. They are merely sending messages between your glands and organs to bring about change…. but they are sensitive. They respond to everything and anything that's going on in your body and FYI they don't really like it when you ignore them, try and drown them in alcohol or suppress them with pain relief medication.

And they especially hate it when you try and override them with fake synthetic wannabe versions of themselves, it offends them, they lose their will to live and sometimes they'll shut up shop all together as a result.

Our poor old hormones have a lot to contend with: inflammation, your toxic lifestyle, infections, your shitty attitude, chemicals from the environment, stress, lack of self-love, dehydration, nutritional depletion, refined sugar, additives. ALL OF THESE THINGS dramatically affect the hormones' ability to do their jobs correctly… to bring about changes in the body which are supposed to make us feel good, keep us fertile, keep our skin healthy and all those other fabulous womanly things.

4. Your environment matters

I'm talking about the world you live in, how it influences your body and the things you are exposed to on a day-to-day basis.

- The foods you consume
- The toxins you apply to your skin, inhale or even consume
- The pharmaceutical medications you use
- The 'natural' yet synthetic vitamins you take daily
- The disconnection you feel from your truth
- The amount of exercise you do or don't do
- How fresh the air you breathe is
- The underlying bacterial, fungal and viral infections in your body
- The tension in your workplace and the financial stress in your life
- The level of fear you experience on a day-to-day basis
- The climate you live in
- How much radiation you are exposed to in the home or workplace
- The level of intellectual stimulation you have.

And all the other many lifestyle choices you make and the level of fulfilment and joy you experience daily. It all counts. It's all affecting your internal environment and your overall health.

5. Symptoms are a good thing

As painful as your period is, as unattractive as your cystic acne is and as uncomfortable as your farty arse in public is….we need to learn to love them! Because this is our body's primary language, it's alerting us to the fact that something is out of balance and needs addressing pronto! When we look beyond the symptoms and recognise it as our body's cry for help, we not only learn to appreciate our body much more and start to build the awareness around the consequence of our daily actions, we're also starting the journey of self-discovery and personal healing.

6. Treat the cause

Our natural human desire to avoid pain teamed with the new age quick fix approach has led to a lot of shoddy botch up jobs which may look good on the outside, but sure as hell don't work so well on the inside. When we don't investigate and address the reason why our body is displaying 'symptoms,' the body will only find another way to let us know it's suffering. Symptomatic treatment is like putting a band-aid over a leaking pipe and expecting it to hold. But the truth is, the problem will never truly be fixed until the pipe is replaced and the reason it was damaged in the first place removed. It's about viewing the body as a whole, not merely seeing it as bits and pieces. Our body works in perfect unison with every single cell communicating with one another. Taking medication to suppress the message your body is trying to alert you to is ultimately the beginning of a long, slow and painful death.

7. There is no magic pill

Healing is a journey. The same journey it was getting to that state of disease in the first place. We must reverse the damage and restore vitality to our cells, which will never be possible with a magic pill. Healing is work, and like the dramatic symptoms that finally grabbed your attention enough to stop you in your tracks and start paying attention to the body, we must be prepared for dramatic change. The innate healing ability of our body is phenomenal, but your body can't do it alone. It needs your co-operation. It needs you to love and value it enough to go within and explore what it requires, to address the causes as to why your body is suffering in the first place and one by one start to undo these damages. You know what they say, "it won't happen overnight, but it will happen" and only when we recognise that health is a privilege not a birthright will we be able to value our bodies for exactly what they are.

8. Prevention vs cure

If we put 20% of our daily effort into making conscious decisions which support our health, we would not need to put 100% of our effort into saving our life upon diagnosis. Prevention will always be a smarter and less painful way to address health. If we choose to ignore the messages our body is giving us over the years, the body must simply speak louder and louder, or rather the disease progresses more deeply until it takes over critical organs and really gets our attention with conditions you simply cannot ignore, like cancer. Ignorance is, after all, a choice.

9. Testing your hormones is largely a waste of time

It's kinda like trying to fill a leaking bucket with water. Testing implies it's the hormones' fault. Fixating on 'proving our hormones are wrong' by measuring something that is continually changing every hour in response to your environment without any willingness to investigate what caused them to go out of whack in the first place, then trying to put them back in order by adding synthetic hormones to try and fill in the gaps. It's inevitable they will fall out of balance again down the track, because you didn't actually address the crack in the bucket first. Pointless really, when you think about it.

10. Question everything

You, my dear, are a very unique and very special individual, and although you share 'common' physiology with every other human, there is nothing common about you. The way your body responds to food, feelings, medicine, technology, treatment protocols and environments is going to be completely different to the next person and this is where you get to tune into you and 'feel' what is right for you.

Look at science, for example. There are a million and one studies proving how beneficial the 'Keto' diet is and equally as many scientific research papers which validate why eating meat, high amounts of fat and animal proteins is not conducive for good health. So, which one is right? Which one is wrong? Neither, because what science fails to address is the profound complex mechanism that you are as a whole – cells, organs, neurological connections, wisdom, feelings, energy and so on. And so, what may be true within a test tube will never be as solid as the evidence your body provides you with daily based on your 'feels'. How your physical body actually responds to different stimuli. We are complex, diverse, incredible miracles and to limit us to the confines of a test tube will never do humans are justice and the phenomenon we are, by following any 'one-size-fits-all model'. Your job is to listen to your body and understand what makes you tick, feel what irritates your system and follow your heart and your head. Do you baby, do you.

11. We are more than our physical body

You have an energy field related to your life force, which is directly influenced by the state of your physical, emotional and spiritual wellbeing. When we're feeling good, well-nourished, hydrated and happy, our life force is strong and so is our vibration, which other living beings can feel when they too are connected. Where you're angry, sad, stressed or your body is full of rubbish and toxins, worn out and depleted, that frequency we emit reduces and our ability to feel our own vibration and communication from our body is diminished.

12. Emotions are your internal guidance system

Emotions aren't always exactly fun to 'deal' with, especially sadness, rejection, fear, anger and all the many other spectrums in between. But there's one thing we need to know about these 'feelings' - they are yet another way our body is trying to communicate with us. Call it your intuition or gut feeling, either way, your body has a very clever way of eliciting an emotion in response to events and situations in your life and we get a pretty clear warning if our choices aren't great for us.

Like that espresso martini at midnight that left you feeling anxious and restless as you stare at the ceiling 'til morning or agreeing to that 'online' date which left your skin crawling because he turned out to be a douchebag like you suspected. Trust your vibes. Your emotions don't lie, and they give us valuable information about our environment and how we are perceiving the world around us. The problem is, most of us don't want to feel any of the above, it's too uncomfortable, so instead we suppress these feelings by distracting ourselves with social media, delicious sugary carbs, binge TV or retail therapy and that signal your body was trying to give you about that situation which we chose to ignore merely gets suppressed. Except emotions carry a vibration of their own; joy being the highest and fear being the lowest, so when we bury those low vibrational feelings deep within the depth of our soul, they tend to fester away, creating a stagnancy and blockage of energy affecting the blood flow and vitality to that part of the body. Until the pressure below the surface becomes too destructive to contain and that emotion expresses itself as a physical symptom, which could be in the form of back pain, hair loss, loss of libido, or even an itchy red rash. Either way, your body will eventually feel the ill effects of negative emotions just as much as it does to the physical harm we place on ourselves through diet and lifestyle choices. If this is a new concept for you, I encourage you to check out Louise L Hay's book, You Can Heal Your life. This is a simple introduction to the correlation between emotions and disease, and I'll go into more detail in Chapter 11.

Now that we've got the lecture out of the way and faced the hard facts we can move on and start making things right. The best part about this whole thing is that your body loves you unconditionally. It doesn't actually care how much you've mistreated it; it's loyal and will heal itself as soon as you start helping it.

I know this wake-up call can feel a little overwhelming. It would be pretty easy from this point to dive under the covers (with a bowl of chips and your favourite 'Rom-Com' movie) and give this book the flick. The struggle is real and maybe you don't believe in yourself right now. Maybe you've been through too much; maybe the pain has been too unbearable. It may feel like there's no light at the end of the tunnel. But I want you to know, I believe in you and sometimes all you have to do is borrow someone else's belief for a while, until you are ready to back yourself.

So, ask yourself this, 'Is what you're doing right now and how you are living your life helping you to feel better?' And if the answer is no, it's time to course-correct. This book is your re-route to hormone harmony. Buckle up and enjoy the ride, you got this girl.

CHAPTER 2

BE A SELFISH BITCH

"It's my body, so it's my choice"
Halo McIntyre (age 2½)

SELF - RESPONSIBILITY

We now live in a world where our poor old hormones are copping the blame for EVERYTHING. And you know what, it's bullshit! I'm probably the first person in history to write a book which defends your hormones, but here's the thing - your hormones merely do as they are told. 'Shooting the messenger' has become the norm. Your skin breaks out and your first response is, 'ah my stupid hormones'. At 'that time of the month' we lose our shit at our mum or boyfriend….it must be your hormones' fault, right? Or maybe your period really hurts, and you feel like death when you're bleeding. Yep, those unruly hormones must be up to their old tricks again. No! Your hormones don't behave badly, they merely react to your internal and external environment.

"I hate being a woman, it's not fair". How many times have you heard yourself say or think that?

If there's one thing I want you to take away from this book, it's this - your body really loves you and ALWAYS has your back. Do you love your body back?

Your body loves you so much it's constantly communicating with you, but it can't speak in words like we'd like it to, it communicates with sensations, things you can feel, AKA symptoms. That headache, diarrhoea, freaking uncomfortable bloating, back pain, anxiety and so on, are all ways your body is letting you know that it's struggling. It's trying really hard to maintain 'balance' within your cells and keep your organs healthy and hence keep you alive, but it's struggling to do the work under some, should I say, 'pretty shitty work conditions'.

Imagine trying to get your work tasks done, but you're drowning in chemicals from the moment you wake up. The multitude of different lotions and potions you put on your skin which absorb into the body, flushing the system with an acidic, nutrient-less latte, your morning 'pills' which the liver has to try and process while it's still trying to deal with last night's takeaway, glass of red and the lack of vitamins and minerals consumed through the non-existent amount of fresh raw food. Oh, by the way, did you drink your two litres of water yesterday? And then there's probably that underlying low-grade bacterial infection in your system, that you don't even know about, that the poor immune system is working tirelessly to keep at bay, the paint fumes you've been breathing in all night in your bedroom if your room was painted within the last 5 years, that toxic (but delicious-smelling) candle by your bedside table, the pollution and car exhaust fumes we breathe in daily, and of course that self-esteem blow you receive first thing in the morning as you take a casual glance at social media. That casual notification check will most often lead to a cascade of stress chemicals which leave you feeling 'meh' about your less than perfect life compared to everyone else's. All this occurs seven days a week and we wonder why our hormones have lost the plot!

We naively punish our body with busy work regimes, huge to-do lists and deprive it of fresh air, filtered water, nutritious whole foods, movement, oxytocin-producing long hugs, deep soulful conversation and good vibes, and wonder why our poor old body is struggling so much.

And you know what, none of this is your fault. We've been misguided and mislead our entire lives when it comes to 'how you should take care of your body'. Naively we've been coerced into believing that everything our healthcare system does for us is truth and the only option. No one taught us anything about diet, feelings and toxins in primary school, so you weren't to know any better. We're not shown how to tune into our bodies and there sure as hell ain't a lot of science being flashed around in the media about the connection between emotional health and physical disease. It's all about the 'latest scientific breakthrough' and what drug you can take to silence the body's cries most effectively. And quite frankly, the lack of awareness and funding that goes into 'health prevention' in our modern-day medical model is appalling. But standing around pointing fingers, whinging about the cracks in the system isn't going to help your health. So, it's up to you to take a proactive stand for yourself and start figuring out your own health journey. And I'm going to show you the way.

Your current health crisis is not your fault, but nonetheless, IT IS your responsibility and if you don't clean it up, no one else is going to do it for you.

If we can step into a place of empowerment and really own self-responsibility, I challenge you to sit with this for a minute. "If your body is hurting, it's kinda your fault." That more than likely is a tough pill to swallow, but I offer that perspective because the key to your freedom, vitality and living in your personal power is about taking responsibility for your body and taking ownership of your own healing journey.

When we are able to acknowledge and recognise that our 'current condition', pains or annoying symptoms are the body's way of saying, 'hey girl, help me out here' that's when we can start to put a plan of attack in place to give the body what it truly needs. That's when we shift from the helpless 'victim' state and into a vibration of hope, giving us a real chance at feeling better. And we can only do that when we are willing to own our body as our own creation.

SELF-AWARENESS

Self-awareness is about truly knowing yourself, being so aware of your feelings and your physical body that you are empowered and in control of your own reality. Self-awareness is recognising you are unique and not getting caught up in worrying about comparing yourself to the girl next door. Having this level of awareness allows us to recognise when we're making decisions which support our highest good or will only make us feel worse, kinda like the game of Russian roulette played when prescribing a pill for every ill. Self-awareness is your doorway to connecting with your soul. It's the ability to listen to and feel your body. It's about trusting your vibe and using your intuition. It's about being so strong in knowing who you are, with a clear understanding of your core values that you never need to question yourself or feel rocked by another person's judgements.

As a human with human emotions, from time to time you will get triggered, but that's when self-awareness gets to kick back in and through the process of self-inquiry you can ask yourself what is your truth in this moment and how do you want to proceed from here.

It's about responding mindfully to stressful situations or nasty comments rather than reacting, AKA… flying off the handle. It's about living in a state of neutrality and acceptance and catching yourself when the negative self-talk kicks in which is merely your deepest fears trying to keep you stuck in your limiting familiar patterns.

Wow, that's heavy, I know, but if you can master self-awareness you become the queen of your own destiny and no smart-lipped 'biatch' is gonna take your throne! The most precious tool that any queen can have is the ability to practice self-inquiry.

On the outside, self-inquiry may seem like a crazy person talking to themselves, yet on the inside it's the stillness and clarity which allows us to listen to our divine wisdom.

Did you know, there's actually nothing anyone else can tell you about your body, that your body doesn't already know. No medical test, intervention or exploratory surgery has anything on the innate wisdom of our body. The only problem is, we have never been taught to listen and that power has been suppressed, most likely for your entire life and generations before.

I get that I'm throwing some new-age 'hippy shit' at you right now and it might seem kinda weird talking to your body, but it's about connecting with your soul and starting to live life on purpose! Your purpose. When we are able to calm the mayhem of 'life' around us and sit in stillness, we get better at feeling and tuning in and listening. This is how we evoke that intuition and inner womb wisdom that may have been asleep but is always willing and ready to be woken should you choose the journey of self-discovery!

To begin playing with the process, we need to practice mindfulness, which is merely pausing and feeling, assessing, listening and processing before we make our next move. It's getting out of those automatic programs we chose to adopt through our upbringing and schooling environment and starting to live life to the rhythm of your own heart.

How often do you give away your power in your day-to-day life, by blaming something or someone else for your situation? What is your story? And do you want to keep living it? We get caught up in how things have always been, making it very difficult to see another way, but this only keeps us stuck in the cycle.

Self-awareness is the perfect companion to self-responsibility because together they create change! Together they are able to shift you out of the deep programming society has handed us, the victim mentality which creates an addiction to our 'diagnosis' fuelled by blame and the inability to take ownership. There is no magic pill, short-cut or secret back door, your journey is to live life experiencing and doing the inner and outer work for yourself, but not by yourself. Healing is a journey and sometimes it's a tough one, but it all comes down to your willingness to flow with the blows of life, surrender, adapt and feel your way forward.

SELF-LOVE

The most important 'self' of them all, yourself! Loving yourself is one of the most important elements of your journey as a human being but for many one of the most difficult to master. We're taught that it's vain to love our self or shameful to put yourself first, but there is a very significant difference between arrogance and self-appreciation and without existing from a place of recognition of just how perfect you are, there simply is no foundation of self-worth and you will never be able to love and care for your body the way it desires.

One of the easiest ways to learn how to love yourself more truly is to consider yourself your own romantic partner or best friend and constantly check in. "Is my behaviour okay?" "How would my lover or friend feel about me treating them this way?" "Would they still want to be in a relationship with me if I constantly spoke to them unkindly, avoided them, had negative thoughts about them or failed to give them any loving attention and nurturing?"

The basic truth to human existence is that you are perfect in your whole natural state exactly as you, only most of us forget this and then set about creating a body and physical features we dislike because we have never given them any care and appreciation. Self-love is mostly about self-acceptance and loving yourself and all that you choose to create. At the end of the day, our body is merely our transportation; we get to choose how we want that to look and how we want to show up. There's so much shame around 'letting yourself go' and equally as much judgement placed on those who opt for surgical procedures, lip fillers and injections, but at the end of the day, all that matters is how you feel about your choices. If you're a Botox queen, then own it, be proud of it and give yourself that creative gift if that helps you to feel better about yourself.

But if you are holding onto any form of self-judgement around your choices, you are still hurting your body. Remember, your physical body is bloody tough, but also very sensitive. It knows when you are hating on it and it feels the burden of personal rejection. You are 100% undeniably beautiful in your natural skin, there is no question of that and the divine feminine in you is creative!

So, have fun and play with make-up, hair styling, new outfits and plastic surgery if that's what you feel drawn to, but do it because you enjoy it, not because you feel inadequate as you are. There's a huge energetic difference between those viewpoints and both will have a different effect on your vibration. Think of your vibration as your invisible ray of light which radiates from your physical body and is a measure of your vitality, inner peace, self-acceptance and self-love.

When we're stuck in negative thought processes, feeling shame, guilt, anger, judgement or anything as equally morbid, our vibrational field is low, and vice versa when we are in a state of happiness and joy! The real magic of this 'vibration' though is the subtle form of communication it provides, interacting with all other living beings. We've all experienced that sinking feeling after chatting with someone who is particularly negative - we quite often feel flat and just as despondent about life as them. But when you surround yourself with high vibrational, excited, positive people, their vibe is almost infectious, and you can't help but feel happy and optimistic. Your vibration is your own creation and it's all based on how you feel.

The higher your vibration, not only do you feel great within yourself, but you will energetically attract more people on the same vibration as yourself and experience more happiness, more energy, more abundance and more self-healing. We've all heard the saying 'laughter is the best medicine', well now you know why. Why is it there's a notable difference between a curvy woman who feels confident and sexy within herself versus a woman of the same shape and size who has a vibration of self-loathing and shame around her figure. You can sense the difference between these women, and I bet you know which one members of the opposite sex naturally gravitate towards.

Your mind might be starting to tick over with your own internal dialogue right about now, 'I'm just not a sexy person, I never have been', the good old ego feeding you the same storylines you've been running your entire life. Well it's time to check yourself before you wreck yourself. "It's your body, you get to choose." How do you want to feel? And if you don't yet know what that feels like, use your beautiful feminine gifts to get creative with your imagination. We create through embodiment and changing our vibration by feeling what we desire. Go on, close your eyes right now and fantasise about whatever you like – it could be a hot session with your secret celebrity crush or a day off from housework to lay on the beach. How does it make you feel? Grab that feeling and focus on it. That's how you create more of what you desire, and the same goes for all elements of your physical body and health, as it does with your mind and what you choose to believe. If you believe you have an incurable disease then guess what, you do. Or you can choose to honour the magnificence of your body and believe that it has everything it needs to heal itself if you just help it out a little. And it starts with self-love.

From this day forth, you get to be as SELF-ish as you like. That doesn't mean shitting all over everyone else, it just means treating yourself with the same amount of love, respect and importance as you do everyone else in your life. A woman who is completely disconnected from her 'self' gives and gives and gives without the ability to receive in return and completely depletes herself, her self-worth and will always become burnt out if she cannot master her own self-love and ability to give to herself.

CHAPTER 3

O DEAR

"In order to change we must be sick and tired of being sick and tired."

Unknown

Welcome to the 21st century, where men get breast cancer and aquatic marine life turn from male to female due to the abnormally high amounts of oestrogen in our waterways.

In the 1600s, the average age women started menstruating was 16 and although that age is not deemed rare in this day and age, it's certainly not the norm. In fact, girls as young as 10 are now beginning their journey to womanhood, and the average age periods begin is just 12½. So, why are we evolving to an era of 'young breeders' so rapidly? Considering we're collectively the most infertile we've ever been as infertility rates continue to soar, I believe it has everything to do with environmental influences and nothing to do with the old 'survival of the fittest' theory of evolution.

There are two prominent things that occur in the lead-up to a woman's bleed. Firstly, it's worth noting that the uterus lining is gradually thickening over the entire course of your cycle, due to the deliberate and precise dance between oestrogen and progesterone. This thickening is a natural process designed to provide nourishment for a fertilised egg should pregnancy occur, but when the egg isn't fertilised following ovulation and the rapid decline in progesterone and oestrogen occur and as a result, the lining of your uterus sheds. 'PMS' occurs when your adrenal glands and liver don't cope with the rapid fluctuation of hormones and as a result your body is sent into a bit of a spin. This is not the time to be condemning yourself for having a vagina and hating on your body for making you crazy. This is a time to go within and nurture yourself and recognise that if you are feeling like shit, you just need to love on your body a little harder. Your bleed is the beautiful symbolic act of releasing, letting go and starting afresh. A menstrual bleed should be celebrated, as it represents fertility and divine feminine gifts which when we're tuned into our cycle become our very own superpowers. More on that later.

The other thing that's going on in the lead-up to your bleed is the increased production of prostaglandins which are actually inflammatory molecules your body deliberately produces in order to irritate the lining of the uterus to initiate the bleed. When your body is already in a pro-inflammatory state, aka you're stressed, toxic, lacking fresh fruit and vegetables and have a chip on your shoulder, your body is irritated in general and therefore already producing too many of these natural prostaglandins, leading to the over-stimulation of the uterus. Hello sharp stabbing cramps or that dull ache through your back and thighs known as period pain! But guess what, if you start connecting into your body and listening to what your body is lacking, or you start having a high antioxidant, anti-inflammatory, cold-pressed fruit and vegetable juice with turmeric and ginger every day, I guarantee you'll reduce your period pain dramatically if you stick at this regime consistently.

And while we're on the topic of period pain, one of the most important messages I want to stress about periods, is that period pain is not normal and not something you just have to deal with. It blows my mind that all journals, blogs or medical papers will all say the same thing about menstruation - "You might feel uncomfortable, irritable and overall in a bad mood. Some of the common menstrual symptoms include cramping, tenderness of the skin and breasts, sudden mood swings, tiredness, headaches and migraines, as well as pain in the lower back". Well they may be freaking common girlfriend, but they sure as hell ain't normal. These 'common symptoms' are your body's way of letting you know that it is stressed and not coping with a natural phenomenon which occurs every month. I can honestly say, that I do NOT experience ANY PAIN or discomfort, breakouts or mental breakdowns (that one's debatable if I'm not following my path) through my cycle anymore and neither will you once you've learnt the secret language of your body!

Oestrogen dominance

Oestrogen dominance is far more than merely the excess of oestrogen in relation to progesterone, despite what Google and Wikipedia will tell you. It's about recognising the role of 'external' synthetic oestrogens and the detrimental effect they are having on our bodies, men included, hence why one in every 1000 men are now developing breast cancer. Scary stuff considering they don't produce very much oestrogen all on their own. So, where is all this oestrogen coming from?

Xenoestrogens are man-made chemicals which mimic and disrupt our natural oestrogen (the stuff our body actually produces all on its own) and can show up in a variety of sources, the most common being hormone replacement therapy, contraceptive pills, rods, injections and implants. But you'll also find them in commercially-raised non-organic meats, insecticide, pesticides, tap water, parabens from your shampoo, soaps, lotions, make-up and other personal care products, BPA (bisphenol-A), Phthalates from soft plastics, the highest source being found in foods wrapped in plastics then heated in the microwave which allows the chemicals to leach into the food you then ingest. But wait there's still more, artificial flavourings such as MSG also have oestrogenic effects on the body, processed forms of soy like 'fake meats' and even your personal care products like tampons and sanitary pads have high amounts of dioxins which too have a disruptive effect on our hormones.

These wayward xenoestrogens are aggressive, and they cause a whole heap of trouble in your body. They cruise around your body seeking out oestrogen receptors (think of receptors like little magnets which fit oestrogen like a lock and key, stimulating the oestrogenic effect on the body). Problem is, they stimulate a far more potent effect than what our naturally produced oestrogen would create, which is why you end up with symptoms such as bloating, breast tenderness, fibrocystic lumpy breasts, low sex drive, irregular menstrual periods, mood swings, irritability, headaches, anxiety, panic attacks, weight gain, hair loss, cold hands or feet, histamine sensitivities, fatigue and memory problems, to name a few.

What's worse, as these foreign fake oestrogens, hog all the receptor sites, there's becomes no need for your body to produce natural oestrogen, which is why so many women have low oestrogen, no sex drive, premature ageing, hot flushes and are being falsely accused of starting menopause at such young ages.

Also, do you want to know why you put on weight around your hips, breasts, thighs, butt, tummy and arms? It's because this is where we store oestrogen. Only because you have way too much oestrogen of the foreign invader style, your amazing body does the only thing it can to protect you from the effects of having high amounts cursing around your body and so it stores the oestrogen away in fat tissue…. hips, butts, things, breasts and tuckshop mama arms! And if your body can't effectively metabolise and eliminate oestrogen from your body, because you have lazy bowels with diminished natural microflora, bad microflora or a sluggish liver, or maybe you've tested positive to an MTHFR gene mutation, well guess what, that oestrogen stays there forever until you do something about it. And you won't be able to lose that excess weight until your body no longer requires those fat cells for storage of oestrogen.

But I haven't even gotten to the most devasting issue of the oestrogen dominance matter yet…the danger your GP or specialist is putting you in by band-aiding the issue with more synthetic hormones and claiming going on the 'pill' will balance your hormones. Newsflash, no it won't! How can it, when you are simply flooding your body with more of the problem which caused the problem in the first place? The current medical form of treatment is to put you on the oral contraceptive pill or use a device known as the Mirena, which is aimed at increasing your progesterone levels to try and match the oestrogen. Notice I said match, not balance. There is nothing 'balancing' about using synthetic hormones to fix a hormonal imbalance. The only way you can EVER balance your hormones is to tackle the underlying issues in your body or environmental influences which have thrown your hormones out of balance in the first place. Remember, balance is your natural state and your body does a damn good job of maintaining it, when we help it out.

Unfortunately, one of the major sources of xenoestrogen exposure that we haven't talked about yet is your bloodline. Awareness around this topic really is only starting to gain traction in recent years, so there's a fair chance ya mama didn't get the memo way back yonder which means you probably inherited oestrogen dominance at the time of conception. If Mum had oestrogen dominance through the pregnancy, your DNA is most likely imprinted with this phenomena, but don't worry you can change this, which I'll explain later.

Stepping back into the blame game for just a minute, back in the old days there certainly wasn't much awareness on the importance of preconception care. Hell, there still isn't much these days, with the painful reality that one in every four pregnancies result in miscarriage and for anyone who's experienced the traumatic process of losing a baby, no matter how pregnant you were or weren't, it's still a devastating loss that can leave painful memories within the womb. But your GP will simply pat you on the back, tell you it's common and send you on your way, claiming there's nothing you can do about pregnancy loss it's just bad luck. Bullshit. Miscarriage isn't bad luck. It occurs because something has gone wrong in the development of your foetus, with the most common reasons being toxicity, hormone imbalances and nutritional deficiency, each which lead to genetic abnormalities and an inability for the foetus to develop normally.

Heavy metals and all these xenoestrogens have a lot to answer for when it comes to miscarriage and the only way to truly protect your child and ensure you have a happy, complication-free pregnancy is to prepare your body for pregnancy by doing a preconception cleanse program and ensuring you are nutritionally sound enough to be able to build a baby from scratch. I think we underestimate just how phenomenal building a human being from just two cells is. It kinda takes effort and if the building blocks aren't sturdy because you're nutritionally depleted and toxic then things don't always turn out the best for bub.

Please don't cut corners when it comes to beginning your family. Too often I receive emails from excited people sharing their news and asking what they should now be taking to support the pregnancy, but unfortunately, they've missed the boat because the 3-4 months BEFORE conception has a far greater impact on the quality of the egg, and the sperm and genetic potential of that child is far more crucial than any supplement you can start taking once you fall pregnant. You know what they say, fail to prepare, prepare to fail. Let's not take human life for granted.

Xenoestrogens have long-term consequences

There's another far greater crime that is made by the narrow-minded approach to 'balancing' your hormones with synthetic hormones and as much as I hate dropping the C bomb, it's a sad and harsh reality we can't ignore. Using the oral contraceptive pill or something alike to mask the signs your body is giving you to let you know it's overloaded with xenoestrogens (painful periods, lumpy breasts, hormonal acne, mood swings, premenstrual headaches and everything else I listed above) is pretty much like dousing a fire with petrol. That slow-burning fire of xenoestrogens is slowly but surely creating a far bigger problem beneath the surface which isn't so easily ignored when it finally emerges from the depths presenting as cancer, breast, ovarian or cervical cancer being the most common among women who have been affected by the synthetic hormones. Your body will work tirelessly to protect you, but if you don't help it out and listen to its cries, and action steps to eliminate the causes of the hormonal imbalance and your exposure to these xenoestrogens, eventually something has gotta give. A tumour, be it a benign cyst or a cancerous lump, is always the result of the body desperately trying to encapsulate harmful toxins which, in conjunction with a suppressed immune system, due to tirelessly trying to contain an underlying resistant infection, systemic inflammation, sluggish lymphatics an overburdened liver and buried emotions we refuse to address.

Loving being a woman

Do you hate getting your period? Have you heard yourself saying 'I hate being a woman it's so unfair what we have to go through with childbirth and monthly bleeding"? Symbolically, shedding your uterus each month is a ritual of releasing and renewing and the cyclical hormonal changes which make this possible are very closely linked with the cycle of the moon, which when we learn to understand the different 'emotional' phases of our cycle we can use to positively impact our lives.

The follicular stage of your cycle occurs on average following your bleed until you ovulate, which could be anywhere from 7 to 14 days depending on your own uniqueness. Think of this stage like the spring; you feel good, your energy and stamina are at their highest, as is your creativity, and you have the motivation, confidence and clarity to start new projects. You genuinely back yourself more, feel more flirtatious and are in a better mood in general as your oestrogen levels are rising, helping you to feel feminine, soft, more easy-going, able to trust your intuition and go with the flow. And with testosterone also rising through this phase, you'll have more self-belief and confidence to try new things, stand up for what you believe in and speak your truth. Yes, girl you are unstoppable.

Ovulation, the summer! Think, 'this girl is on fi-ya', your most expressive self emerges and your ability to communicate and connect with others is unstoppable! This is your most social stage of the cycle where you are most attractive to others intellectually and physically and will find yourself winning arguments you never thought you could and manifesting your desires like a mofo! Your 'inner mama,' whether you have children or not, appears and you see the best in all those around you whilst igniting your innate nurturing qualities to help others and feel good about it in the process. Oh, and with your hormones peaking, this is also when your libido peaks each month, so if you're feeling more sexual than ever….go get it girl, just remember it's also your most fertile time of the month.

Autumn, post-ovulation, also known as the pre-menstrual phase or luteal phase of your cycle is the time when your progesterone, oestrogen and testosterone are all declining following ovulation and you will feel your most withdrawn. This is not a bad thing though, it's a time to slow down, go within and listen to your intuition. To stop doing so much for others and simply nurture yourself and listen to your body. If you feel 'crazy' emotional through this stage of your cycle, it's most likely because your intuition is at its highest and your body wants you to know something.

Self-enquiry is your friend through this stage, so ask yourself why you are feeling so irritated, irrational and downright raging. Where are you out of alignment in your choices, where are you not living by your own values, where have you been led astray? Your bullshit detector is at its highest in this phase so it's not a bad thing if people around you are annoying you. Are you just seeing them for who they really are while the veil is lifted? Tune into those gut feelings - what are they trying to tell you? Is your body secretly mourning as you live a life that isn't what you truly desire, within your career, community, hobbies, relationship or personal beliefs? When we understand this stage of the cycle is designed to help us slow down and go within and we stop trying to be how we are during our first stage of the cycle, this can be an extremely powerful stage of insight and personal growth, rejuvenation and regeneration.

Period time, the winter, the time to retreat and hibernate. The day you start bleeding is day one of your cycle, it's the time of releasing all that new wisdom you acquired through your pre-menstrual phase and reflecting. This is a time for serious self-care. If you experience period pain, quite often this is your body grieving or protesting. Where did you not love yourself enough this last month? What do you now need to let go of that no longer serves you?

Making peace with your period and learning to love it is going to be one of the most important things you do! You can spend this 30-40 year period of your life in disgust and resentment about the fact 'it sucks to be a woman' or you can surrender and embrace the beauty and magic that comes with being a woman. I bet you can guess the ones who struggle more with endometriosis, cysts, fibroids and all kinds of gynaecological dysfunction - those who have not made peace with their female bits and beliefs around the divine feminine woman.

And for all you non-menstruating mamas and post-menopausal queens, you still have access to these cycle superpowers, it's just going to take a little deeper tuning in to recognise where you are within that natural cycle without the period happening.

Earlier I casually dropped 'buried emotions' as a cause of disease. Now is probably a good time to explain exactly how that works. Painful emotions are uncomfortable, and the majority of the population would do whatever they could to avoid them. The problem is, emotions are kinda like symptoms and you can't just ignore them and cover them up with pills, because even though in the short term they may feel out of sight, out of mind while you distract yourself with that online shopping addiction, grab a serotonin high by stuffing yourself full of chocolate or numb yourself with alcohol, negative emotions are also another way your body communicates with you, often prompting you to make a change, be that in your personal life, romantic life, career or values and perceptions of the world.

Painful emotions such as fear, sadness or guilt should always be considered an internal compass to navigating you away from choices which do not serve you. Then there are emotions such as grief following the loss of a loved one, which although is completely out of our control, if we don't take the time to sit with these feelings and process them correctly, they will quite often leave behind an emotional scar which impacts the state of your physical health. There's plenty of scientific research which validates the physical effect that stress, and suppressed emotions have on the body. Look at unchecked anger and the effect it can have on blood pressure. Suppressed grief very often manifests as a disease within the lungs, trauma from sexual abuse is likely to create disease within female reproductive disorders, back pain the result of feeling alone and unsupported, and feelings of shame and low self-worth will very often affect our physical appearance by means of acne or skin rashes.

Quite often, the women I see who are suffering the most severely with diseases of the womb, ovaries or vagina have deep suppressed feelings of shame, personal rejection and anger which they have not made peace with.

MY STORY

I remember being mortified after spotting my first pubic hair at around age 11. I cut it off, only to see another ten return days later! Then a couple of years later I got my first period and felt even more shame. For some reason I had a lot of irrational beliefs around being a woman and fearing what that represented to the opposite sex, as I certainly didn't want any attention from boys at that age, or to be thought of as a slut. Somewhere along the way I had decided that being a woman 'too early' was something to be ashamed of. Clearly as a 13-year-old virgin who hadn't even kissed a boy or had a boyfriend, my perception of the word 'slut' was somewhat warped but nonetheless it certainly represented a disconnect which was always going to catch up with me eventually and most likely related to why I experienced such traumatic 'hormonal' issues later on.

I remember telling my mum that I got my period, and although she was warm and supportive, she harmlessly made the observation that I was much younger than my older sisters who didn't start menstruating until 14 and 16 respectively, which made me feel like even more of a 'slut'. What was wrong with me? Why was I different? This was a theme that played out frequently in my adult years, causing me much separation and pain, until I learnt to love my body and dissolved the underlying fears, misguided beliefs and self-judgement around what being a woman and a beautiful, sexual woman meant.

Protecting Yourself From Oestrogen Dominance

Action

- Clean up your beauty routine – opt for organic, chemical-free makeup, toothpaste and deodorant
- Same goes for your cleaning regime – throw out your nasty chemical household cleaning products and go green
- Stop using tampons and disposable pads and replace these with medical-grade silicone menstrual cups and organic cloth pads or 'period knickers'
- Get a BPA free, stainless steel or, even better, glass water bottle
- Get a good quality water filter in your home
- If you suffer from period pain – try natural anti-inflammatory herbal products like Turmeric and essential oils
- Make peace with your period. Revisit the day you first bled and explore what emotions that bought up for you.

Check out the Balanced Babes resource section for my favourite picks www.balancedbabes.net/resources

CHAPTER 4

THE PROBLEM WITH THE PILL

"Truth, the pill that everyone wants but can't seem to swallow."

Anonymous

Bad Science Vs Good Science - where'd all the common sense go?

In 1965, the Supreme Court gave married couples the right to use birth control. This was after many years of this method being considered illegal after it was first created by Margaret Sanger in 1916 when she opened her first birth control clinic but was later jailed for 30 days after being considered a public nuisance for her 'promiscuous' invention. It wasn't until 1972 after a change in formulation, due to questions surrounding its safety, that the oral contraceptive pill became legally available to all women regardless of their marital status.

The new age inconvenience, your bleed

Fast forward the clock 50 plus years and the number of teenage girls on the birth control pill has jumped by 50% in the past decade in the US alone, according to a study by Thomson Reuters, with 29% of teenage women (13-18) filling prescriptions for oral contraceptives in 2009. So, why are so many young girls, who are not even sexually active, reaching for this pharmaceutical drug which has vast short-term and long-term implications?

I'd like to first point out the difference between a side effect and a consequence. I feel that this has been a play by the pharmaceutical industry to naively dumb down the potential risks associated with using synthetic hormones which have steered women away from their own responsibility to understand what is actually occurring within their body and why. And I'd like to just casually point out that are no 'side effects' caused by the pill, merely reactions based on what this drug does to your body. Until we take the time to recognise that all of our choices come with consequences, we are still giving away our power and not making conscious informed decisions with our own best interests at heart, falling back on the belief that it is our GP's responsibility to take care of us, whilst assuming he knows every single thing about your health including your family history, lifestyle choices and how your body specifically will respond to chemical changes brought on by the pill.

Yes, I'll be honest, if I had it my way, I'd be telling everyone to turf their prescription hormones in the bin, but realistically I understand most of you can't do that. It's convenient, it provides peace of mind surrounding unplanned pregnancies and for a lot of you, you're probably not even experiencing any major noticeable symptoms that you can't deal with. The real issue I have with the pill is more so about its incorrect use, being prescribed to mask underlying symptoms which irresponsibly divert women from looking for the real cause of their hormonal discomfort.

Here's a list of reported consequences which have occurred among women using the oral contraceptive pill or other forms such as implants, rods or injections based on reactions women have experienced over the years.

- Breast tenderness or swelling
- Mood changes, including mood swings, increased anxiety or symptoms of depression
- Nausea, vomiting, bloating, stomach cramps
- Irregular bleeding or spotting between periods
- Changes to menstrual periods
- Decreased sex drive and loss of libido
- Nipple discharge
- Increased hair growth
- Loss of scalp hair
- Pigmentation including freckles and darkening of facial skin
- Headache, migraines (including new cases or worsening of symptoms)
- Changes in weight or appetite
- Vaginal itching or discharge
- Problems with contact lenses.

Furthermore, various clinical trials studying the safety and efficacy of the drug over the years have revealed it is linked with a higher risk of breast cancer, increased risk of blood clotting, heart attack and stroke, gall bladder symptoms and disease, increased blood pressure and benign liver tumours. And for those of you who did take a proactive response to your prescription, here's a few things you won't find written in that little product insert from your pharmacist. Ignorance is bliss, until it happens to you and then you're faced with the turmoil and anguish of wishing you had have known better or had more body awareness to recognise the symptoms unfolding, allowing you to intervene sooner rather than later. When we know better, we can do better.

Low libido and complete disconnection from your body

Some of you will experience PMS on steroids while using the pill; a very distressing out of body experience. This is a scary place to be in, for you and those in your path. You can see yourself losing control, as if the real you has temporarily checked out and is watching from above as you lose your shit at the kids or your lucky man, but there's nothing you can do to stop yourself, because in that moment, you have zero control. Then, within minutes, shame, denial, sadness and exhaustion set in. It really is a heart wrenching low to reach.

Synthetic hormones are more or less foreign invaders and absolutely in those moments of rage, it is these irrational, thoughtless monsters which have taken over and possessed your thoughts and actions. But until you take back your power by saying no to their antics by seeking an alternative method of contraception, the buck stops with you, so is the responsibility of the warfare you're creating in your world.

MY STORY

When I was 17, I put myself on the pill for the first time. I remember telling my doctor it was because I was distressed about the state of my acne, which wasn't all that bad, because I was too embarrassed to admit I'd just become sexually active. Within weeks of starting, the foreign invader went to work on my body and completely messed with my entire chemistry, leaving me feeling completely crazy. I was so irrational and emotional; I could barely even hold a conversation with my poor mum without it ending in tears or rage (sorry Mum). The internal feeling of angst, feeling completely disconnected from my body is something I will never forget. It was as if everything I ever feared was being awoken inside of me, all of my insecurities came flying to the surface, my organs felt like they were crawling inside of me, I was crippled with anxiety and I even had suicidal thoughts, which was completely out of character for me and something I had never experienced before.

Believe it or not, I consider myself one of the lucky ones because I was able to work out that this had only started when I began the OCP, Dianne-35ED. So, I went back to my GP who told me what I was experiencing was quite normal. He then gave me a new prescription for another very common pill, Levlen ED. Although things were not quite as 'crazy,' I still didn't feel myself and couldn't deal with the intense mood swings, crying one minute, raging the next, and completely numb the rest of the time. I was then recommended Yasmin, which was a lower dose pill and I felt dramatically better, so I persevered with this product, completely oblivious to the very gradually increasing size of my breasts, rounding of my face and candida infection building within.

After nine months I had a shocking wakeup call via the scales gaining 5kg, fighting thrush infections on and off, and looking in the mirror not really liking or recognising the person I saw anymore. I looked bloated, my eyes were lifeless, and I had no desire to have sex with my boyfriend anymore, which was ironic considering that was the reason I started taking the pill in the first place. I realised I was completely disconnected from my true feminine essence and my self-esteem had taken a huge knock through the process. Because when you don't truly know yourself, what are you really living for? If you don't know what makes you happy, how can you experience joy? Without the ability to 'feel,' how do you know what you're passionate about? Disconnection is having no idea what your values are, no sense of purpose or belonging to something outside of yourself and no appreciation for the simple everyday things like human interaction. This is when addictions and substance abuse will kick in, desperately searching for something outside of ourselves to help us feel something, even if it is a temporary binge on sugar.

That disconnection is created when, like a robot, these synthetic hormones start to possess our bodies. That numb feeling gradually gets worse as we lose touch with ourselves then start to pull away further and further from our romantic partner. Intimacy and affection become insignificant to the artificial highs we can achieve through wine, chocolate, retail therapy or self-deprivation.

I believe the oral contraceptive pill plays a huge role in many relationship problems, due to the loss of intimacy, women feeling misunderstood by their partners, reduced libido and the vacancy within your heart as your body is ransacked by synthetic hormones completely affecting your ability to flow from your innate natural cycle.

Let's take a look at how the OCP actually works to prevent pregnancy. It works by preventing the release of an egg (ovulation) during your menstrual cycle. It also makes vaginal fluid thicker to help prevent sperm from reaching an egg (fertilisation) and changes the lining of the uterus to prevent attachment of a fertilised egg. If a fertilised egg does not attach to the uterus, it passes out of the body. Our divine feminine wisdom becomes suppressed shutting down our intuition, which I believe has contributed to why we've become a generation so disconnected from the magic of menstruation and connection to our divine feminine wisdom that more and more women are opting to skip their monthly bleed altogether. Unfortunately for many, 'that time of the month' has evolved to be a time which is dreaded by many due to the harshness of their painful cramps, severity of mood changes and heaviness of their flow, making it not only a damn right nuisance, not being able to wear white, the awkwardness of swimming and the sheer debilitation of pain and emotional outbursts. If you're reading this and even the thought of your period rolling around each month makes your ovaries ache, then it's crucial you seek help, to heal your painful periods, and you do this holistically. Continuing to suffer like this, convincing yourself it's normal and just something you have to deal with or worse, manipulating your pill prescription to skip the 'hormone-free' sugar tablets is setting yourself up for disastrous long-term consequences with your fertility and placing you at an alarmingly higher risk for breast, ovarian and cervical cancer.

In 2015, 1365 new cases of ovarian cancer and 857 cases of cervical cancer were diagnosed in Australia alone, with a subsequent 1197 combined deaths in 2016 from these 2 types of cancer the following year.

In 2015, 16,852 women and 145 men were diagnosed with breast cancer in Australia. One in every eight women will be diagnosed with breast cancer in Australia. In 2016, 2976 women and 28 men died of breast cancer in Australia, with all statistics taken from the Cancer Council Australia.

Exposure to elevated levels of natural or artificial female hormones has been noted as increased risk factors in each of these cancers.

Maybe you've done your time and you're no longer menstruating but as a mother with your fresh new perspective on the issue at hand, you get a chance to have these conversations about what periods represent – health, vitality, fertility and the right of passage to womanhood, something that should be celebrated and honoured. If we can adequately prepare young girls for what is ahead and share with them the wisdom of their cycle, framing the experience as an initiation to womanhood and not merely an 'inconvenience that females unluckily have to endure while men get off scot-free'. I highly recommended paving the way for period acceptance by having a mini celebration with your daughter when she reaches menarche by taking her to lunch, purchasing her a new outfit or anything which creates excitement and helps your daughter to feel excited about reaching this milestone and becoming a woman.

For ways to deal with painful periods and hormonal changes please check out the 'Treatment Protocols' section of Balanced Babes. https://balancedbabes.net/treatmentprotocols

Helping girls to understand the deeper meaning of their monthly cycle and the privilege of bringing life into the world and ensuring that their understanding of a normal period is one that is pain-free and symptom-free is the only way we can start to change the culture around women's health and bodily functions.

Bio-identical hormones - close but not close enough

This is an issue which blatantly points out the vast difference between 'natural' and holistic, which for the most part, many don't seem to understand. In my opinion, this confusion is what really threatens the safety, effectiveness and future of natural medicine because the difference is very profound.

In the case of bio-identical hormones, we're still missing the mark. More and more women are opting for a 'safer' more natural alternative to the aggressive and risk-filled synthetic hormones associated with HRT (Hormone Replacement Therapy) but this poses challenges of its own. Bio-identical hormones are, for lack of a better term, a 'more natural' approach, created from extracts such as yam and soybean, but what we need to understand is that they still have very unnatural synthetic ingredients and that approach to balancing your hormones is still very far from a holistic approach, because we are still ignoring the very reasons why this woman is experiencing 'hormonal' discomfort in the first place.

Think of it this way. You've got a bucket and the goal is to fill it with water. But your bucket has a crack in it. Using 'hormone replacement therapy' or lathering your body with creams, gels, patches or shoving it up your hoo-ha, be they synthetic or natural, using 'bio-identical' forms of hormones is like trying to fill that broken bucket up with water. No matter what, you've going to have to keep running the water continuously if you want that bucket to stay full while it has a leak in it. A holistic approach to the same situation would be stepping back, observing the bucket, identifying why the problem isn't going away, mending the bucket by addressing the cause of the leak and then allowing the bucket to do what it is meant to do. Hold water. Mission accomplished.

Well-meaning doctors and Endocrine specialists have a legal obligation to provide a solution for patients problems but are unfortunately letting women down, by addressing their symptoms through a narrowed approached, merely addressing the symptoms in a quest to rapidly relieve symptoms. Which as a woman suffering from debilitating hot flushes, mood swings, excessive bleeding and so forth is pretty damn appealing. But if we do not identify, heal and strengthen the foundation of these women's bodies they will be left reliant on these dangerous synthetic hormones long-term, increasing their risks of heart disease, stroke, breast cancer and so forth, or eventually that hole in the bucket will just get bigger and bigger and the symptomatic relief won't work anymore.

Don't get me wrong, there will always be situations where a fully holistic approach, addressing the causes of the hormonal imbalance is not going to suffice, in cases where glands and other body parts have been removed through a hysterectomy etc. There are also rare cases where people are not born with certain glands and will therefore never be able to produce the hormones naturally. And yes, the holistic approach is a slower one and it takes more work on the woman's behalf, but it will always be the safest and most effective in the long run as it will shine a light on all areas of ill-health and prevent these minor cracks becoming bigger 'diseases' in the future. If you want to live a long, healthy life and you don't wish to succumb to the classic 'old age' conditions; Dementia, Alzheimer's, Parkinson's disease, Glaucoma, Diabetes, Osteoarthritis, Hypertension and Cancer, your best bet is staying as far away from pharmaceutical band-aids and learning how to listen to your body then giving it what it needs to thrive with holistic supportive therapies from healthy eating, self-care, connection with nature, natural cleansing and body therapies. Our life choices and how we live our life while we are young is dramatically a direct correlation to the quality of life we will experience in our years beyond 60. Remember, every action has a consequence and it's rarely ever an immediate one.

Some of you may feel defeated, having tried a 'natural' approach in the past, whether that be an optimistic attempt at self-prescription from your health food stores or booking in to see a qualified therapist, but if all of the major factors which contribute to hormone havoc, as I've outlined have not been sufficiently addressed, you were never going to make any decent headway with your symptoms by treating at a surface level, be that with the use of synthetic drugs or natural remedies.

Using the pill and synthetic contraception safely

If using a form of synthetic hormonal contraception is the only suitable method for you and your partner, then it's important to support your body through the process to prevent side effects and long-term hormonal imbalance, especially issues which can arise when you decide it's time to transition off birth control and start planning a family.

From a physical level we must support the body from the burden these synthetic hormones place on the liver as well as the risk of oestrogen dominance which builds up in your body if you are not effectively metabolising these hormones out of your body, which is unfortunately inevitable with long-term use.

As a primary consideration, ensuring your elimination organs are strong and healthy is a must. Moving your bowels a minimum of twice a day, drinking two litres of filtered water every day to flush your kidneys, lymphatics and skin of impurities and toxic by-products. Partaking in a gentle seven-day liver cleanse program should be done at least every four to six months to prevent the backlog of hormones in your body and allow the liver to keep up with the processing of your hormones. The Balanced Babes 'Babe Cleanse' is a free option which can be found on the Balanced Babes website at: https://balancedbabes.net/treatmentprotocols

This is an easy to follow guide which includes a liver cleansing eating plan and recommended daily cleanse activities to give your liver a spring clean and maintenance.

Another factor which cannot be ignored with the use of synthetic hormones is the impact this medication has on your nutritional status. A report from the World Health Organization (WHO) points out the influence of oral contraceptives in causing key nutrient depletion of folic acid, vitamins B2, B6, B12, vitamin C and E as well as the minerals magnesium, selenium and zinc. Long-term deficiency of these nutrients will have a significant impact on immunity, fertility, mood and general wellbeing due to their vast requirement in common biological processes within the body in the manufacture of neurotransmitters, immune cells, digestive secretions and hormone production. If you choose to use hormonal contraception, supplementing to support these depletions should be considered a first-line approach by clinicians according to the WHO.

The Pill and thrush

Also known as Candidiasis, an infection caused by *Candida albicans*, which has the most pronounced effect within the vaginal canal presenting with itching, redness and a thick whitish-yellow discharge at its worst can often become more common among women using the oral contraceptive pill. To say the pill causes this infection is a little far-fetched, however, the use of synthetic hormones certainly has an effect on our natural production of hormones which can make your system more susceptible to thrush, namely through the imbalance in the natural vaginal flora.

With the depletion in 'healthy lactobacillus bacteria' from within the uterine canal due to reduced natural secretion of oestrogen, this opportunistic infection may present. What is also important to note, candida albicans is not the only culprit which grows out of control and is always present with an underlying strep infection, which will most likely go undiagnosed and untreated through the traditional treatment prescribed through conventional medicine, anti-fungal applications, which allows for the strep to continue to run havoc until correctly addressed. Check out Chapter 7 for more details.

Looking beyond the physical manifestations of synthetic hormones creates the need to understand that with the replacement of your natural hormone production, which is completely derailed with the use of the pill or any other method of administration, is the inevitable suppression of your own innate 'natural' cycle, which comes with consequences of its own. This disconnect from your natural cycle quite often leads to a loss in our ability to tune into our intuition, which the tsunami of 'fake' hormones railroading our natural production of neurotransmitters eliciting their own emotional response. This will quite often result in heightened reactions to situations or feelings of numbness as we become more and more robot-like at the mercy of the dose of oestrogen or progestin you've administered on that particular day.

Recommended resource: Passion to Purpose- Reclaiming your Personal power, online learning course. An online program which equips you with the tools to reconnect with your values, passions and purpose. Check out https://balancedbabes.net/passion-to-purpose/

Contraception alternatives

So, what do you do instead? This is the million-dollar question. Unfortunately, I don't have the answer you probably want to hear. When it comes to safe, effective natural contraception, there really is no magic 'safe' pill. Although there is a large variety of methods men and women can explore, each requires concentrated effort on your behalf researching and understanding how to use them. In my opinion, the male condom will always be the first port of call for contraception due to its effectiveness and the fact that it also protects from sexually transmitted diseases.

Beyond this there are various methods which include intimately understanding your cycle, mucus changes, temperature and charting to have a clear understanding of when you are ovulating, however I do warn that it's quite normal for a woman's cycle to change by a few days here and there based on the moon cycles and who she is keeping company with. It's not uncommon for women to sync their cycle with other women they are spending time with. And then of course there's always the health of your partner's semen which will determine how 'active' his swimmers are inside of you for how long.

Charting and understanding your cycle is definitely something all women should practice as it will help you to understand how and why you are feeling but in terms of contraception the good old male condom will always be your best bet and if you think the rubber is uncomfortable, trust me they've come a long way since 3000 BC when condoms were made out of fish bladders, linen cloths and animal intestines!

PART 2

'THE 7 STEP HORMONE HEALING SYSTEM'

Let's be honest, you can Google any symptom you like and you'll no doubt find a blog with the top 10 herbs, nutrients or natural solutions to make that symptom go away. Handy hey? No.

You are probably reading this book because you tried that, and it didn't work. Maybe I'm being hasty, maybe you tried it and it worked for a little while or it worked at first but then the moment you stopped popping your 'natural' pills it all came crashing down again….your symptoms that is, the mood swings, the acne, the painful periods, the hot flushes, the weight gain or whatever else you were trying to fix with your Google search.

Don't get me wrong, I'm team Google, especially when it comes to 'natural medicine'. I'd way rather you try your hand with natural approaches than turn to your GP for a quick chemical fix. But here's the thing.

THERE IS NO MAGIC PILL.

There's no quick fix and let me tell you why. Because your body speaks. It communicates through 'symptoms'. That headache, those dark bags under your eyes and that painful bloating is your body's way of letting you know something's up.

And your body wants you to listen. Your body doesn't want you to silence it with a pharmaceutical prescription or a natural remedy, it wants you to work with it and address the reason why you're feeling shitty.

I've been stressing this since Chapter 1, but in case you're still not down with the 4-1-1, your body is awesome, it's smart and it totally has your back. So, if something feels bad, it's a sign your body isn't responding well to the way you're living your life. You know those double shot espresso coffees, red wines, lack of exercise, polluted drinking water (or maybe chocolate ice-cream is your jam), the point is you are experiencing uncomfortable symptoms because something you are doing or exposing yourself to is hurting your body and your body wants you to start taking better care of it, so you can both keep living your best life.

If you want to heal something like swollen breasts, anxiety, or annoying eczema/dermatitis, the same rules apply. TREAT THE CAUSE. I'm not meaning to yell at you, I'm just trying to make it clear, you will never solve your health problems by throwing them under the rug or suppressing the symptoms with a pill, be it chemical or natural , if you ain't addressing the deficiency, infection or toxicity (the only three reasons why you get sick in the first place). The symptoms won't go away or it will only come back again.

There are just no shortcuts. And that, my friend, is why I created the 7 Step Hormone Healing System. So, you can get the job done right, once and for all.

This system is for anyone who is experiencing anything uncomfortable in their body on a regular basis, be it reoccurring UTI's, feeling tired and run down all the time or being diagnosed with something a little more hectic like endometriosis, PCOS or an auto-immune condition. This system is also for anyone who wants to start taking a proactive approach to health and wellness. We all know conditions like breast cancer, heart disease and diabetes exist, and here's where you get to choose. Keep doing what you're doing, because right now you're still able to get away with it or learn how to listen to your body and buffer the consequences of living life large by understanding what your body needs.

You don't have to be 'sick' to benefit from the 7 Step Hormone Healing System. Everyone has hormones and everyone's hormones are under threat if you are living a standard lifestyle. So, think of the recommendations in the following chapters as not only cures but preventers.

I'm not asking you to give up your guilty pleasures and stop having fun. I'm all about BALANCE (remember I'm a self-confessed chocoholic).

Let's just learn how to listen to our body while it's still whispering, gentle nudges, and not screaming at you through pain you can't ignore.

Let's learn the art of self-care and make it fun, so we can keep enjoying the finer things in life, the over-indulgence, the wild nights out with girlfriends, your favourite beauty hacks (chemical hair straightening right here and proud of it) and the 'sometimes' foods. You are human, you came here for a human experience – to enjoy all those incredible human senses – touch, taste, smell, sound, and the other ones I can't remember - but the point is we're here to have a good time, right? Let's just also make it a long time. The choices you make in the first 30, 40, 50 even 60 years of your life dramatically affect the last 10-20 years of your life. We all know elderly people who are suffering, hurting day in and day out, struggling with their dementia and popping pills for every ill, with each new prescription causing yet another side effect that they need another drug to suppress. It's devastating. And we all have a choice right now, to take care of our body and choose to address the cause of our illness rather than enter the deadly merry-go-round of prescription medication that is very difficult to get off once you start on that road.

Over the next seven chapters you'll be getting up close and personal with your body, learning how to prevent common ailments and how to heal them by understanding what they actually mean. You'll have a complete step-by-step actionable 'treatment protocol' for healing your body of debilitating conditions and take back control of your body! No more giving away your power and relying on someone else to 'fix' you. Let's go girl!

How to use the 7 Step Hormone Healing System

There are two parts to healing your body; addressing the physical imbalance and the **Spiritual Shape Up**. You cannot heal without the delicate balance between spiritual/emotional and physical healing, and that's a fact.

For the physical element of your healing journey, all instructions are laid out per chapter with additional instructions which can be found at the Balanced Babes website. https://balancedbabes.net under the resources or treatment protocols sections. This includes additional videos, product recommendations and further detail into your healing protocols.

Additionally, you will need to download the 7 Step Hormone Healing System Guided Meditation, which you can do so at the website. https://balancedbabes.net/resources/balancedbabes-meditation/

To effectively heal your body and tap into your female superpowers, you will need to get yourself a journal so you can 'journal the journey,' because journaling your experiences is just as powerful as the physical work you'll be doing to heal your body. Writing is a powerful way to get out of your analytical mind and start to tune into what you are 'feeling' as opposed to thinking. This is a crucial tool in learning to understand the messages your body is giving you and to allow you to reconnect with your soul.

Before each Journaling the Journey session you undertake, we recommend you listen to the guided meditation with a set of headphones to completely block out outside noise and really go within. To really enhance the rate that you connect with your body, I recommend getting in the habit of listening to the short meditation daily and journaling for at least 15 minutes.

Meditation is something I resisted for a long time. I was 'too busy' and I didn't know how to silence my thoughts, so I just didn't bother doing it. Well, the truth is, you don't need to silence your thoughts, you actually need to listen to them and understand them. Observe the thoughts that are coming up.

Use guided meditations in conjunction with the journaling.

While sitting in meditation ask yourself the prompted chapter questions, stop and listen. You will receive the awareness as your body starts to talk to you and the answers pop into your head. Maybe as memories or visions. You may hear clear voices in your head, or you may just start to feel things. This awareness will continue to come to you over the following days, once you start listening, the more your body will reveal and quite often even show you through sensations and symptoms.

Commit to this practise daily, because it's going to be the most important thing that you can do to reconnect with your body and understand what your body needs to thrive from day to day! Don't stress if it doesn't feel natural or you're not getting the answers straight away, meditation is a practice after all.

And remember, EVERYTHING is easier with support, so don't be shy, share your journey and ask your questions in the Balanced Babes Facebook Support Group which you can join here: https://www.facebook.com/groups/balancedbabes4life/

CHAPTER 5

GIRL, YOU'RE A HOT MESS

⟵————————⟶

"A wise girl knows her limits, a smart girl knows that she has none."

Marilyn Monroe

Picture this. It's 6:30am and your alarm has just irritatingly started squawking at you. You're so tired, there's no way you want to get up, but you've got a job to be at and a household to organise. Your head feels foggy, you're exhausted because you stayed up way too late lost in your Insta feed, the white light of your phone completely throwing your circadian rhythm out, affecting the production of melatonin and balance of cortisol. In fact, your whole body's exhausted. You haven't had enough sleep. You've been burning the candle at both ends, running around with work commitments, trying to be a wife and a mum, probably not fuelling your body with optimal nutrition or enough water and so your body is in a state of stress. But the only way you know to get yourself going is to grab a coffee. And so, you proceed to blast yourself with that acidic fuel, throwing your blood pH out of whack and demanding the adrenal glands to produce even more cortisol to wake you up, because you have no choice but to keep going. Sound familiar?

Rush, rush, rush, go, go, go. Your body is now in a state of distress, your nervous system is wired, making it difficult to actually think clearly as you thrust into the 'fight or flight' mode. You become reactive, snapping at anyone in your path who doesn't appear to be helping your cause. You're dehydrated, but too 'busy' to recognise you're thirsty and besides you don't have time to think about yourself right now. Your poor adrenal glands are in overdrive!

There are 101 things going on and while depriving yourself of the basic necessities your body would love upon waking, their job is now just to keep you alive! When operating from the flight or fight mechanism, you become disconnected from your body and completely unable to listen to the messages your body is trying to give you.

You've probably heard it before, adrenal fatigue. In this fast-paced 21st century lifestyle where Wi-Fi is as common as oxygen, more and more people are struggling with this common phenomenon, adrenal burn out. The only problem is, when we're busy, we're not necessarily present in our body and that's bad news for our adrenal glands. Self-awareness goes out of the window, making it very difficult to take responsibility for listening to what you need right now.

The truth is, it's actually your hypothalamus which is responsible for maintaining your body's internal balance, providing the link between the endocrine system and the nervous system, but it's your adrenals glands that do the heavy lifting, which is why they are so sensitive to burnout.

Think of these two glands as workhorses constantly on alert ready to release adrenaline and cortisol the moment the hypothalamus detects change. Your adrenal glands are the first to respond through their production of 'stress chemicals' to initiate balance back into the body when our internal environment is 'stressed'.

Stress is anything that has the ability to threaten your internal environment and the smooth workings of the body. Stress could be that morning coffee you've just drowned without having any water first leading to dehydration and adding to the livers workload. Stress is your boss giving you a hard time because you haven't met a deadline. Stress is looking at the bank account and seeing that you don't have enough money to pay the bills this week. Stress is gaining weight around your organs, which leads to inflammation. Stress is not getting enough vitamins and minerals in your body. Stress is anything which threatens the internal balance of your body.

This is where the 'flight or fight' response comes in, a mechanism which your body cleverly crafted to protect you from dangerous situations. When this system is activated by stress, adrenaline and cortisol are produced, signalling increased glucose availability to your muscles to allow you to run away from predators and elevated glucose to your brain, to help you to think on your feet. For many, there's an additional mode, the 'freeze' response which will often kick in when you're so overwhelmed by stress and fear that you actually just freeze. This reaction isn't so good for survival but I'm sure you can see where that one plays out in your life from time to time.

The problem is, this 'fight or flight' reaction has become our default go-to mechanism because people are living in constant stress, never truly calm or relaxed. With so many things on our to-do lists, trying to achieve more, trying to do the whole 'boss babe' work from home mum thing, we're putting more and more pressure on ourselves to perform, which is overloading our adrenals. These little powerhouses are doing their best to keep you on top of your game but without adequate rest and restoration, adequate nutrition and enough relaxation balance to calm your nervous system we are depleting our poor adrenals, giving rise to a new age pandemic, adrenal fatigue.

The Three Stages of Adrenal Fatigue

	Stage 1 'Adrenal Activation'	Stage 2 'Adrenal Distress'	Stage 3 'Adrenal Fatigue'
Energy Levels	Generally good energy levels	Energy levels fluctuate from high to low, typically experiences a '2nd wind' in the evening after a 3pm slump	Low energy levels consistently throughout the day
Nervous System	Heightened awareness of heartbeat, some anxiety	Anxiety and often panic attacks	Depression or low mood
Sleeping Habits	Minimal sleep disturbance, some difficulty falling asleep due to a 'busy mind'	Bouts of insomnia, sometimes feel 'wired but tired'. And lay awake for hours or wake frequently through the night	Sleeping regularly and for long periods but never feel refreshed
Eating Habits	Over-reliant on coffee, energy drinks, sugar, alcohol or other stimulants	Feel the need to eat carbohydrates more regularly or will not feel satisfied/full	Commonly eat a lot of processed refined sugars and take away foods due to lack of energy but also have developed a lot of food intolerances, especially to gluten and dairy

	Stage 1 'Adrenal Activation'	Stage 2 'Adrenal Distress'	Stage 3 'Adrenal Fatigue'
Immune System	Rarely get colds or sick in general	Starting to get more frequent colds, 2-5 colds per year or other infections i.e. urinary, chest, sinus, tonsillitis, thrush	History of past viral infection as well as frequent infections ongoing
Body Weight	Typically healthy weight range, although a tendency to store excess fat around mid-centre	Weight changes, difficulty losing weight, starting to put weight on more easily especially around the mid-section	Can be severely underweight or overweight but typically starting to store more body fat all over the body
Persona-lity Traits	Constantly on the go, overactive mind, high achiever, rarely sits still, needs to feel productive	Memory and concentration starting to struggle. More frequent emotional outbursts of anger and irritability	Lack of motivation and energy, feelings of hopelessness, sick of being sick and not feeling yourself
Bowel Health	More prone to loose motions, especially when stressed or anxious	Bowels fluctuate between loose to constipated	More prone to constipation
Thyroid Health	TSH levels within the classic reference range of 0.5- 5	TSH levels started to increase as thyroid health is beginning to become affected	Underactive thyroid, high TSH levels, with thyroid antibodies starting to rise

BALANCED BABES

	Stage 1 'Adrenal Activation'	Stage 2 'Adrenal Distress'	Stage 3 'Adrenal Fatigue'
Physical Symptoms	Tendency to an internal feeling of shakiness, butterflies in the tummy	Sweaty hands, hair falling out, skin starting to break out	Hair loss Skin rashes Food intolerances Bloating
Blood Sugar Regulation	Typically, can't go too many hours without eating without feeling irritable, headachy or shaky	Insulin resistance starting to form	Loss of appetite, regular nausea
Oestrogen Status	May experience shorter menstrual cycles due to low progesterone levels. May experience spotting throughout the month	Periods starting to become irregular, with longer cycles	Very irregular periods, often with absence of a period for extended periods of time
Dream Recall	Can wake with vivid dreams or nightmares	Irregular dream recall	No dream recall
Cortisol Production	Excessive, high amounts	Irregular, but levels beginning to deplete	Cortisol deficiency, adrenals unable to secrete adequate amounts
Muscular Health	Twitching and occasional muscle cramps	Muscles becoming tired, weak and sore with some cramping and eye ticks	Tired, sore aching, weak muscles

	Stage 1 'Adrenal Activation'	Stage 2 'Adrenal Distress'	Stage 3 'Adrenal Fatigue'
Cellular Fluid Levels	Fluid retention around monthly cycle	Noticeable fluid retention around face, arms, thighs, belly, chest	Systemic fluid retention

This is not detrimental to your health long term, but it certainly makes you feel uncomfortable, and if left untreated, it's going to progress into stage two. That's when things get more serious. That's when you're going to see changes in your menstrual cycle. You might start to skip a period, or you might get your period more often. You'll definitely see some changes in your weight. This could be weight loss or weight gain, depending on how you are metabolically programmed. It starts to suppress the immune system. Whereas in stage one you'll find you never, ever get sick because it's like everything's working in overdrive, including your immune system. With the 'panic' that occurs in stress, your immune system too responds to the increased adrenaline, which is great in the short term, no infection can pass, but of course it can't sustain that sort of firepower long term, especially as the elevated stress starts to deplete your nutritional stores and before long, you'll progress into stage 2, adrenal exhaustion.

The immune system becomes more fragile because it's burnt out and worn out. Your energy levels will start to decline. Your emotional needs won't be feeling as stable. You will be feeling more flighty in terms of irritability and moving into things like depression and low mood. Your sex drive will be out the window, and if you don't check yourself before you wreck yourself in this stage, you will eventually progress into stage three which is known as chronic fatigue. Unable to get out of bed, plagued with constant infections and underlying opportunistic viruses start to build strength in the presence of your weakening immune system. In stage 3, periods may disappear or become irregular, the thyroid function struggles and your mood continues to decrease. The brain fog due to viruses and the heavy metals they secrete becomes overwhelming. Teamed with your lack of energy, it's difficult to break this cycle once you reach this level of dysfunction.

Having the self-awareness and ability to pick up on the signals our bodies are communicating is crucial. When our workload's getting too much and we're not keeping up. That anxiety, that insomnia, those headaches, that anxiousness. It's a sign that you're not in balance and your body wants you to slow down. It's a sign that your body needs more nourishment and restoration and less of the stimulants. These symptoms experienced in stage 1 are warning signs as opposed to 'annoying body dysfunctions' and if we take the time to listen, feel and intervene early on, we have the ability to prevent disease ever-progressing any further. The problem is, most of us are too loyal to our agendas and completely ignore our bodies, using stimulants like caffeine and sugar and even alcohol to help you keep forging on, but essentially, you're drawing on vital energy reserves that your body relies on in chronic illness. Herein lies the danger of suppressing your symptoms with pharmaceutical medicines or even using natural therapies to avoid discomfort. If you're not addressing your body as a whole, you can completely miss your body's warning message.

Exercise, weight management and adrenal fatigue

Exercise is a hugely misunderstood factor concerning adrenal health, especially when it comes to weight management. We've been conditioned to think the more exercise, the better the results, as we become fixated on achieving that ideal body. But unfortunately, if you're already worn out and depleted, high-intensity exercise or too much of it in general becomes yet another thief of those already waning vital reserves. Exercise has amazing health benefits - increasing circulation, stimulating white blood cell production, supporting lymphatic tissue, stress relief, boosting mental clarity and so on, but if you are already depleted and you're flogging yourself to work out while you are exhausted when you should actually be resting, exercise can become detrimental to you. And the only way to assess this, is to check in after a session. "How am I feeling? Do I feel completely wiped out, and need to rest for the next couple of hours before I can do anything else, or do I feel energised after a workout?"

When it comes to weight loss, if your body is in any one of the different stages of adrenal dysfunction, meaning you've been in fight or flight mode for an extended period of time and your body is in survival mode, it will intentionally retain weight. With its aim, to keep you alive, it switches to a fat-storing agenda, not a high fat-burning mode and so no matter how much exercise you perform, if your body is stressed, it will only store more fat and you'll merely be exhausting glucose supplies through your training sessions, actually driving your body into a deeper state of stress.

The type of exercise you are doing also matters. If you are experiencing symptoms from any of the stages you may need to adjust your exercise regime to a more restorative form, like yoga, walking, Pilates or so on, something which does not stress your body by expecting you to maintain an extremely high heart rate over long periods. In some cases, you may even need to temporarily break from exercise, supplementing your regime with infrared sauna's or lymphatic massage, which allows your body to restore, whilst still receiving the immune-boosting, lymphatic and circulation support you would through raising your heart rate with exercise. Listening to your body requires self-enquiry every day. When you start to stop and listen, you'll get better at trusting your intuition and understanding what is best for your body on a day-to-day basis. Check in daily.

The same applies to dieting. That same programming that 'calories in vs calories out' is the only basic equation for weight loss is very outdated and directly influenced by the state of your adrenal health. In an adrenally stressed individual, rapid calorie restriction diets will only precipitate the stress. The body will respond by slowing down your metabolism even more to preserve for the famine. In these cases, low carb, high fat, high protein diets are the worst thing you can do as your body has temporarily prioritised carbohydrates as a lifesaving fuel, aka a quick accessible form of glucose to fuel your brain and muscles. Quite often I see women in the clinic whose diets are actually perfect, but there's no way their body will shift any of their excess weight due to the state of stress the adrenals are in.

The other thing we have to keep in mind is the effect of our adrenal health on our emotional wellbeing. If your body is in a flight or fight reaction, it's going to be defensive, and so is your outlook and attitude. You're going to be a lot more sensitive to things around you, and that could respond in outbursts of anger. It could also result in retracting, becoming more depressed and withdrawn from society and the people around you. When in a hyper state of stress, this has a roll-on effect onto your neurotransmitters, overstimulating their actions which can often lead to over-excitement of the nervous system, leading to symptoms of insomnia and anxiety.

Throughout my twenties, I had a full social life and didn't much like the idea of staying home alone. I was out and about five nights a week, working full-time, and studying additional courses. Late nights and loads of fun, but I was adamant that if I was going to live that sort of lifestyle, I had still need to honour my body, but without the ability to truly listen to my body back then, my idea of honouring, aka disciplining my body, was actually hurting myself more. It didn't matter what time I got home from the clubs or my nightlife, I was up on the beach at 6am every single morning going for a run before work, because I thought that I had to be dedicated and disciplined to exercise or I would put on weight. The problem was, that exercise session was further detracting from my rest period.

So, when my life and priorities started to change, I decided to stop drinking all alcohol and eating so much sugar; two stimulants which my body had adapted to rely on heavily through this sleepless period of my life. When I stopped these, completely emptying my vital reserves, I literally had nothing left in my tank. So, by removing these stimulants without first repairing and restoring my health, my adrenal glands literally crashed and burned! In crisis mode, I developed hot flushes and my thyroid became underactive with no nutritional stores to keep it functioning. My liver, which was so overloaded with toxins from the high intake of alcohol over the previous five years, now started to detox. But because it wasn't functionally optimally it wasn't able to properly metabolise the toxins it was now releasing and in conjunction with a congested colon and sluggish bowel movements, these toxins were released out of my skin instead, resulting in cystic acne on my back.

Essentially my body went into a form of hibernation. Without the life force to sustain itself, everything started to slow down. My digestion became sluggish, I struggled with the cold, my mood was flat, and I had zero energy. The only way out of this was to ride the wave of exhaustion and rest, restore myself nutritionally, repair my damaged tissues and allow my body to heal.

Healing your body

Restoring adrenal health is absolutely the first stage of the 7 Step Healing System, because cellular repair simply does not occur while in survival mode with all bodily resources going into the fight and flight reaction to keep you alive. Weight loss, the menstrual cycle and fertility become the lowest priorities, as supporting another life is not sustainable at this point. Your body is defending itself and the only way to reverse this is to provide it with nourishment, rest and address all immediate threats to survival.

Step 1 - Addressing Adrenal Health

✗	✗	✗	✓	✓	✓
STRESS	STIMULANTS	SYSTEMIC INFLAMMATION	SLEEP	SELF-CARE	SUPPORT

The 3 R's for recovery

Restoring your adrenal health is completely different from one person to the next. Some people may only need a week of slowing down, taking a few days off work, reading a book instead of going to the gym, restricting themselves from late night social media, eating fresh fruit and vegetables, having cold-pressed juices daily, soaking in some relaxing Epsom salt baths. The other person may need to be in that state of restoration for up to a month or even longer depending on how long they've been exhausting their vital reserves and how long they've been depriving themselves of good health.

Rest

If you have no energy at all, you need to do some serious work on slowing down, tuning in, calming yourself down and doing some restorative work on your body. Only then will your adrenal glands be able to restore their normal function. This is a vital step which cannot be ignored and can often take discipline to action. A big part of resting involves learning how to say no, making your own health and wellbeing your first priority and giving less out. This is a particularly difficult skill to become used to as society as a whole condemns anyone for putting themselves first, branding them as selfish, but if we do not first take care of ourselves, we don't have the resources to take care of anyone else without depleting ourselves, which will always lead to resentment whether you are consciously aware of it or not.

Restoring the adrenal glands is always a slow and steady approach and healing takes time and largely involves sleeping more. I know you're rolling your eyes at the thought of resting more, thinking, "Well I don't have time to rest," but if you don't rest, your body will find a way to make you rest, and a deeper illness will force you to stop. Letting go of control and the expectations you've placed on yourself is paramount. Allowing yourself to utilise company sickies or calling on more help or babysitters for your kids may be something you have to prioritise in the short term. Listen to your body, what does it need from you right now?

Relaxation

Get out of your head. Find your happy place. This is more than just laying around on the couch, watching Netflix completely checked out, it's taking steps to learn how to relax your mind and body. It's learning how to centre yourself and go within to remain calm even when chaos continues around you. It's also about protecting yourself from toxic people, friends who drain you and identifying where you need to put boundaries in place. Checking in daily and asking yourself how you can best spend your energy today and what will help you to feel good versus what will suck the life out you.

Sometimes this is not an easy process, but you need to learn how to feel. One of this program's most important components is to learn how to feel and we do that by stopping, connecting with our breath, silencing the noise around us, and just feeling your body. This helps us to become more aware of our energy or vital force. Feeling the energy connecting every single cell within your body communicating with the organs, all syncing to create life. When we become too caught up in 'doing' we lose the ability to 'feel'. The practice of mindfulness gifts us the ability to think before we react and allows us to make choices based on our body's messages and highest good. From this place we get to live life on our own terms based on what feels good and honours our own body. Adrenal exhaustion is very much a disease of trying to please others and draining yourself in the process.

Repair

Our incredible body has its own innate healing mechanism, but it can only tap into this when we are out of the stress response. To initiate repair at a cellular level our body requires nutrients from whole foods, adequate hydration from filtered water, superfoods and restorative herbal medicines to nourish it and allow it to heal your cells. It is very important to focus on giving back to your body and never put yourself on any calorie-restrictive diets or heavy metal detox programs which will only deplete you further. While in this stage of recovery, building your vitality and increasing your energy levels is the primary goal and this is what you will use to identify when you are able to take on the next hormone healing step.

Recovering from stage 3 adrenal fatigue

When you hit rock bottom, suffering adrenal fatigue and chronic exhaustion, there's very little energy or motivation available to make the necessary lifestyle changes to recover. Starting slowly by giving yourself simple tasks which you believe you can carry out will not only set the wheels in motion for change but will instil more confidence in your own ability to care for yourself again, which is a vital part of recovery. Half the battle is always mental. With each addition of a new 'healthy practice' your motivation will grow and the desire to work on your health becomes addictive. It's very important to practice patience and kindness with yourself, as your journey to recovery will always have bumps along the way.

One of the most common things clients report is their difficulty to maintain commitment and dedication to their healing, and the easiest way to counteract the 'falling off the wagon' fear is to implement the healthy actions around your current lifestyle. If you need to bend the rules a little to make something more achievable in the beginning, then do it. Work out what is realistic within your current commitments and level of health and implement as much as you can. Trying to do too much too quickly will quite often lead to overwhelm and result in doing nothing at all, so it comes down to meditating for just 5 minutes a day instead of 20 or getting 5 serves of veggies compared to your usual intake of just one serve a day, even if that falls short of my recommended 10 serves, you are still winning. Doing something will always be better than doing nothing at all. Choose small, obtainable goals, don't set yourself up for failure from the beginning. Remember we're not just healing your body right now, you're teaching yourself new lifelong healthy habits, so make them enjoyable until you are conditioned to these activities being a part of your normal daily routine.

Aligned Action

Stage 1 Intervention
- Drink 2-3 litres of filtered water daily
- Increase your intake of foods high in magnesium and vitamin C to fuel the adrenal repair

Magnesium-rich foods:
- Almonds
- Avocado
- Black beans
- Cacao (dark chocolate)
- Cashews
- Edamame
- Kelp
- Molasses
- Quinoa
- Parsnips
- Pumpkin seeds
- Soy products organic non-GMO
- Spinach
- Sunflower seeds

Vitamin C rich foods:
- Blackcurrant
- Broccoli
- Cabbage (raw)
- Capsicum (red)
- Citrus fruits
- Kiwi fruit
- Papaya
- Parsley
- Pineapple
- Potatoes
- Strawberries

- **Choose a relaxation remedy.** This could be meditation, a massage once a week, lying down and listening to a podcast or music, or zoning out to Netflix in the short term. As long as you're physically stopping, silencing your mind and resting your body.
- **Rest.** Implement a 20-minute 'rest' as many days of the week as you can - whether you sleep or not, just ensure you switch off.
- **Eat 3-5 pieces of fruit daily.** There is no such thing as too much fruit sugar, it restores adrenal health and fertility. Just eat it or juice it.
- **Sleep more.** Aim to be in bed earlier, even if it's just 30 minutes earlier than usual. Unplug from social media no later than 8-9pm and wind up screen time in general, including work.
- **Adrenal restorative herbs.** Including all or some of the following: Rhodiola, Rehmannia, Ashwagandha, Licorice, Siberian Ginseng, Lavender.

Stage 2 Intervention

- **Eat 10 serves of vegetables daily.** Work your way up but make this your goal. Aim for 3 serves at brekkie, 3 serves at lunch, 4 serves at dinner. Choose smoothies and plant-based breakfasts, not heavy processed cooked meals in the mornings which burden on the liver, creating more stress on the adrenals.
- **Mineralise your tissues by correcting key mineral deficiencies.** Traditional mineral formulas such as Ayurveda shilajit, colloidal minerals, trace minerals, humic and fulvic acid etc. are great sources.
- **Start to eliminate 'stressors' from your life:** alcohol, sugar, caffeine, your dickhead boyfriend, jerk boss, energy drinks, your addiction to adrenaline (stop watching scary AF movies).
- **Get more organised** so you're not frequently in running late 'go-go-go' mode.
- **Add anti-inflammatory foods to your diet:** Turmeric, ginger, seeds, fresh fruits and vegetables.
- **Replace your coffee with restorative herbal teas:** Licorice, holy basil, ginseng root, matcha green tea (still high in caffeine), chamomile, peppermint, orange peel, jasmine.

Stage 3 Intervention

- **Create a sacred space.** This is a beautiful space that you can create in nature or your home that feels relaxing to you. Somewhere you can sit and just 'be' for 5-10 minutes to unplug, restore and regenerate. Choose an environment that helps you feel peace and calm.
- **Essential oils:** lavender, bergamot, chamomile, ylang-ylang, rose and vetiver to calm the nervous system.
- **Epsom salts bath or foot soak to restore magnesium levels.**
- **Exercise.** Based on your adrenal dysfunction, determine the right style, frequency and intensity of exercise for you. Tune in following a session - do you feel restored or wiped out? Scale it back accordingly and check in each day.
- **Support thyroid health.** Natural iodine from Kelp, Seaweeds, Ashwagandha, Selenium, Zinc, Magnesium, Goji berries, B12.
- **Limit exposure to Wi-Fi.** Turn phones to flight mode at night, turn home internet off while sleeping. Source protective electromagnetic frequency equipment for your home.

Spiritual Shape-up

Listen to your 7 Step Hormone Healing System Meditation with earphones on then answer the following questions in your journal. Remember, just let the pen flow, whatever comes to your thoughts write it down, even if that means getting side-tracked from the questions, they're just prompts. You may like to address just one question per day and spread them out over a few weeks.

Journaling the Journey
- **Why am I so uptight?**
- **What are my biggest fears and worries? Are they warranted?**
- **What am I afraid of?**
- **Am I being a drama queen?**
- **What is it that's stressing me out?**
- **What are my biggest worries? Are they even warranted?**
- **Who am I living my life for?**
- **What are the things I go for when I'm stressed?**

For example, when you're stressed, do you go for coffee or do you go for chocolate? Do you go into avoidance? Do you go into a rage? Know your reaction so that you can start becoming more aware of it and put a plan into place for it.

CHAPTER 6

RELEASING YOUR SHIT

"In the process of letting go you will lose many things from the past, but you will find yourself."

Deepak Chopra

Are you full of shit? You probably don't think so, but the truth is, the average human has around 2kgs of stagnant fecal mass stuck inside their colon. That's a lot of crap. In fact, did you realise that a true, healthy bowel empties its contents within 45-60 minutes after ingesting each main meal, three times a day and anything less than that is actually considered constipation. Yep, that's right, we should all be shitting at least three times a day to keep ourselves regular. How many times do you go potty a day?

It seems to have become the norm for people to only move their bowels once a day, but you'd even be surprised how often I see women in the clinic who are lucky to even go every couple of days and unfortunately there's a lot of serious consequences from not moving your bowels frequently enough.

Sorry, I know it's a 'shitty' conversation, but this is one of the most important stages of the 7 Step Hormone Healing System because if we are not moving our bowels, we're not emptying the waste out of our system and our body becomes toxic, which has a direct impact on our hormone health. You see, your bowel wall is a permeable membrane, which means the contents can move in and out into the bloodstream quite rapidly. So, if waste material is hanging around too long due to sluggish bowel activity, toxins recirculate back into your system where your liver has to start the clean-up process all over again.

Our poor livers are already completely overworked and that's not even if you live a clean lifestyle with so many environmental factors we're exposed to out of our control. And since your body always has your back and keeping you alive is its goal, the liver will always prioritise more severe toxins like dangerous chemicals, heavy metals, viral residue and so forth, which means your good old hormone metabolism gets put to the waste side; well your reproductive hormones anyway.

Because we are producing hormones all the time, to maintain healthy hormone balance, these hormones need to be removed, recycled and metabolised from your system constantly, which just isn't possible when your liver is already struggling. That stagnant waste inside the colon and bowel of partially undigested food, hard to break down meat and other animal products then starts to rot, providing the perfect festering environment for parasites and harmful bacteria to thrive in. This produces even more toxic waste, creating an acidic environment and causing general havoc with the normal cellular functioning of your body.

All that toxicity begins to overflow from the bowel, spilling out into the systemic circulation where it then comes into contact with your major organs, placing further stress on your system, affecting your mood, digestive health, and continuing to burden on the liver. Think of it this way, when your bowels aren't evacuating effectively or completely, a toxic cesspool of waste is constantly seeping into your bloodstream. Now that's enough to make anyone sick over a long period of time and a great reason why you should be embracing colon cleansing!

The other reason your bowel health is so important for hormone health is because the digestive system, which is just an extension of the bowel, houses your gut microflora which is the complex community of microorganisms that live in the digestive tract and is crucial for overall health. And although this area of study is still very new and still not completely understood, we do know that these beneficial bacterium play a vital role in nutrient metabolism, hormone metabolism, drug metabolism, maintenance of the gut lining and gut mucosal barrier, immunomodulation in terms of the regulation of immune responses, which is largely important when it comes to fighting infections, allergies and the role of auto-immune conditions, as well as protecting against pathogens and foreign invaders. This friendly bacteria also plays a huge role in keeping your hormones in balance, so when the bowel environment is so toxic and overrun with pathogens and bad bacteria that the beneficial flora cannot thrive, hormonal problems such as oestrogen dominance becomes a huge problem.

Now you may think that this doesn't apply to you because you happen to move your bowels two or three times a day. But the question is, are you moving your bowels effectively? Are you completely evacuating? And are you moving your bowels naturally? That is, is your body naturally bringing on a bowel motion through the natural involuntary muscular contraction known as peristalsis which gently moves contents through the digestive tract or are your bowel motions being triggered by irritative foods like gluten containing grains, coffee, dairy, alcohol or sugar? These inflammatory foods have an abrasive effect on the digestive tract, creating a reflex spasm effect, which quickens bowel transit time, which is not a healthy way to initiate a bowel motion as it dramatically affects your body's ability to break down and absorb the nutrition from your food.

I see it all the time, people getting caught in the 'fake fibre' trap exclaiming, "if I eat Weet-Bix my bowels move regularly but without a 'high fibre' cereal breakfast I can't go in the mornings." Unfortunately, highly processed cereals and grains are not what nature intended for your bowels. Weet-Bix is actually very high in gluten, an inflammatory protein, which due to many reasons has now mutated in a way that humans are unable to digest effectively and causes loads of inflammation within the digestive tract, leading to leaky gut syndrome. With this in mind, your bowels are therefore not operating via their designed mechanism, which means they're not truly eliminating effectively, which over time leads to lazy bowel syndrome. The lazier your bowels become, the less efficiently they evacuate, which leads to a build-up of fecal mass that sticks to the colon, hardening over time, forming a mucoid plaque which perpetuates the cycle of toxic overload in the body, creating that perfect breeding ground for parasites as well as severely affecting your ability to assimilate nutrients. But the problem doesn't stop there. In 2015, 15,604 people in Australia alone were diagnosed with Colon cancer, an issue that is largely influenced by this toxic, sluggish, inflammatory, infestation phenomenon we have going on within the digestive tract.

And like every common inconvenience, the medical industry formulated a pill to solve every problem - laxatives. But the problem with laxatives, other than the fact they are following suit and completely ignoring to address the cause of your 'blockage', they are disengaging the bowel and overriding the need to initiate peristalsis, resulting in a lazy bowel.

Poo is one of those subjects that many people don't like to talk about. It's stinky and somewhat awkward. It's really important that we restore our bowel function and create an environment where that microbiome can flourish. In fact, if you don't clean up your bowels, that toxic mess moving through your body will lead to more than just hormonal imbalances. A toxic colon will inevitably lead to acne or other skin conditions due to the body now having to force these toxins out an alternative elimination organ. It dramatically affects our mood and creates that 'shitty' feeling, and due to the backlog of toxins building up in your body, the liver stops being able to burn fat effectively, leading to weight gain and is often the cause of unexplained nausea. Doing a colon cleanse is non-negotiable. I know it's not particularly fun but if you want to have healthy skin, lots of energy, a waistline that you love and healthy, balanced hormones, cleansing the toxic mess out of your colon is unavoidable.

Colon cleansing

Picture a fish tank full of fish that hasn't been cleaned for months. There's a thick residue of fish 'waste' that's building up on the sides of the tank. If you wanted to clean the tank, you wouldn't just replace the water and magically expect the rest of the tank to scrub itself clean. You must first remove the old dirty scum from the sides of the tank. It's the same when trying to clean up your body. If you want to clean up your congested acne covered skin, scrubbing away at the surface will have no effect if you do not address the source of the toxicity coming from within your dirty filter, aka your body. Cleansing the colon is like replacing the filter and allows for your body to eliminate toxins more effectively. If you want longevity, boundless energy, healthy skin and balanced hormones, embracing colon cleansing is something that you need to do. There are lots of variations available, so it's important to find something that works for your lifestyle, but the main thing is that you give it a crack and do it at least twice a year, every single year. I recommend doing it a minimum of three times for a minimum of three days at a time, but I'll share with you 2 different ways so you can explore which is going to best suit your lifestyle.

There are three major things you need to consider as part of a colon cleanse.

Cleansing companion

The most important element of a cleanse is the cleansing product you use to clear the colon. It's important to use something safe, natural and free of irritative laxatives. Many colon cleansing products rely on the use of magnesium oxide which will nonetheless bring on diarrhoea, but it does so by inflaming the colon wall, not cleansing its contents. That mucoid plaque is like rubber and even if you are moving your bowels 2-3 times a day, I guarantee you, you're not budging that plaque, so choosing herbs which can effectively soften and release this gunk is crucial. High amounts of fibre are paramount to moving the mess out of your colon. Think of your cleanse formula as something which will act as an internal broom, sweeping through and scrubbing out the stuck residue. Psyllium husks, yucca root and oat stem are great fibres which work well in conjunction with prebiotics from slippery elm, passionflower and licorice, which soothes an irritated digestive tract. A good formula will also include gentle anti-parasitic herbs such as black walnut and pumpkin seeds to help combat the parasite infestation.

Diet

What you consume through your cleanse period directly influences the effectiveness of softening that mucoid plaque so that it can be loosened and removed. There are variations as to what you can consume while cleansing, which you will need to choose based on your lifestyle and experience with cleansing, but at the very least you must stick to a plant-based diet and avoid animal products in order to give the digestive system a break and reduce the load on the liver. Even better is sticking to raw food. Raw food brings lifeforce to your digestive system, with the natural enzymes assisting with the electricity to spark that peristaltic movement. However, the most effective way to rapidly remove the mucoid plaque over a short duration is to perform a juice fast while cleansing the colon.

The thought of going without solid food can be a tough task to get your head around, but it is a short period of time, requiring as a little as 2-5 days for maximum impact. Drinking nothing but fresh cold-pressed juice gives your digestive system a well-deserved break. It stimulates natural digestive secretions and most importantly softens that mucoid plaque that's been stuck in your intestinal lines for probably years and throws the liver a lifeline.

Hydration

High water intake is paramount! This is to ensure the increased fibre you are consuming with your cleanse can actually move through your digestive system and support the filtering of your system, allowing toxins to flush out through additional elimination channels through sweat, urination and even exhalation. While cleansing you want to aim for a minimum of four litres of good quality filtered water each day.

Maintaining bowel health

Enemas

Now I know you don't want to hear this, but enemas ARE LIFE! Personally, I do them 4-5 times a week and if done right they can definitely help you maintain a healthy weight, vibrant skin, balanced hormones and boost your energy levels. You're probably rolling your eyes and thinking I'm a crazy woman for suggesting that you stick things up your butt but trust me there is a method to this madness. Enemas are a really effective way to maintain a clean, clear colon and fast-track the elimination of toxins on those occasions you feel like over-indulging! Remember, I'm a chocoholic, it's my one vice and I'm able to get away with it, without breaking out in acne or putting on weight because my body can effectively eliminate the toxins before they infiltrate my system, because I'm helping the liver out. And FYI, an enema after a night out drinking is always a sure way to reduce your hangover the next morning!

Essentially, a basic enema is designed to flush out waste from the bowel or lower colon, however when we administer therapeutic agents into our enema bag, the game starts to change a bit.

There's a lot of information out there about coffee enemas, including fear-based accusations, but like anything, if done responsibly with some common sense, can provide a healing effect in the body. Coffee enemas were made popular by the work of Dr Max Gerson who dedicated his medical research to the treatment of cancer and other chronic conditions. He saw coffee enemas as a means of detoxifying the body of "poisons" living in the tissues. Coffee enemas have been reported to have the following benefits:

Repairing digestive tissue
Cleansing the liver
Improving blood circulation
Increasing immunity
Helping with cellular regeneration
Relieving digestive issues, such as frequent constipation, bloating, cramping and nausea
Improving gut health
Improving low energy levels and moods (such as fighting signs of depression)
Boosted energy cell production
Enhanced cell growth

The therapeutic action of coffee enemas is thought to come from a compound in coffee called cafestol palmitate which is said to stimulate the activity of an enzyme called glutathione S-transferase, which opens up the bile duct in the liver, allowing for an increased release in bile from the liver to break down food components and other chemicals and improve digestion.

Personally, I'm a fan of coffee enemas, but you've got to also understand the impact they have on your body. They're an amazing way to stimulate detoxification, but when eliminating chemicals from the body, the action of transforming toxic metabolites into water-soluble substances which the body can safely eliminate requires antioxidants, amino acids and vitamins to support the process. Which means we can deplete ourselves nutritionally by overstimulating liver pathways or create inflammatory damage in the system when there are not enough available minerals to support the detoxification process.

We must also remember that coffee is irritative by nature, having a very drying effect on our mucus membranes and a taxing effect on adrenal health due to the caffeine intake, so I do recommend keeping coffee enemas to a maximum of 1-2 times per week, replenishing any lost electrolytes and minerals in the process and supporting your system with adequate hydration and rest afterwards.

If you like the idea of keeping your colon clean - which I highly recommend - there are many other therapeutic solutions which are more subtle and safer to do more frequently. Try lemon juice or organic turmeric powder to support detoxification, apple cider vinegar (highly diluted) to tame a candida overgrowth, garlic for parasites or chamomile tea or aloe vera juice to soothe an irritated, inflamed bowel and support digestion. You can even use essential oils in enemas using antimicrobials oils such as oregano and frankincense, but always remember to make these solutions up with filtered water and always do your research in regard to dilutions and doses of your therapeutic agents.

Enema success
There are a few things you need to know about enema safety. Firstly, don't believe everything you read on Google. Perforating your bowel is highly unlikely, just be gentle upon insertion and don't use anything really abrasive in your solution that would 'burn' or ulcerate your bowel. As long as you're using filtered organic products in realistic quantities, you can't do any harm. Would you drink one cup of apple cider vinegar on its own? No, then don't put it up your bum. That's the basic rule of thumb to remember when selecting your remedies, if you'd drink it, you can enema it!

Enemas and constipation
A lot of people worry about becoming too reliant on enemas, and yes that is a risk if you're doing them wrong. Never use an enema to bring on a bowel motion; always ensure you use your bowels naturally before performing an enema. If you are congested and can't move your bowels, you really need to work on getting that bowel function happening again before you start relying on enemas to bring it on because that approach is no different to using laxatives in terms of the dependency that forms. If you start doing the job for your body the body will start directing its attention and energy elsewhere. See the tips below for supporting natural bowel activity and treating constipation.

Doing an enema should not be painful, but because the bowel is lined with muscle, you can experience uncomfortable cramps. Start slowly in terms of how much liquid you administer and listen to your body in regards to when it's time to release. Don't force yourself out of your comfort zone too much. Being a muscle, it takes work training it, so just be gentle and remember to breathe. Enemas take practice, they get easier over time.

Colonic irrigation

Also known as colon hydrotherapy, this is a more specialised practice which requires a qualified therapist to safely administer water and other therapeutic solutions through the anus to gently flush the colon.

The flow of pressurised water in a controlled environment helps to remove built-up congestion from a toxic colon and assists the proper function of your body's organs by restoring your gut and colon health, as well as overall wellbeing. Compared to self-administered enemas, the machine allows for water to cleanse the entire colon rather than just the descending colon, which can be more or less relaxed depending if you prefer the assistance of someone else.

Retraining a lazy bowel

If you're someone who's been sluggish for a really long time, you're going to need to perform a bowel retrain protocol. Although this is non-invasive and easy to do, it does take time and consistent effort. This is about re-establishing the brain-bowel connection and re-firing the neurons to the smooth muscle of your digestive system to signal peristalsis. Now, you might have already succumbed to the fact you're a 'naturally constipated' person because you've 'been like this since I was a little girl.' Well girlfriend, I can't urge you enough to change that story if you want to avoid hormone imbalances in the long term, including how well you handle menopause when the time comes. Ensuring your bowels are moving effectively every single day is key to preventing diseases of toxicity later in life. We know that issues like cancer are largely developed due to excess toxicity within the body. A tumour is essentially like a little rubbish bin that your body creates to encapsulate the dangerous waste to protect it from your organs. When you remove the trash regularly, you prevent your body from becoming a deadly dumping ground. Check out the Balanced Babes bowel retrain protocol here: www.balancedbabes.net/bowelretrain/

Step 2 - Combating Chronic Colon Congestion

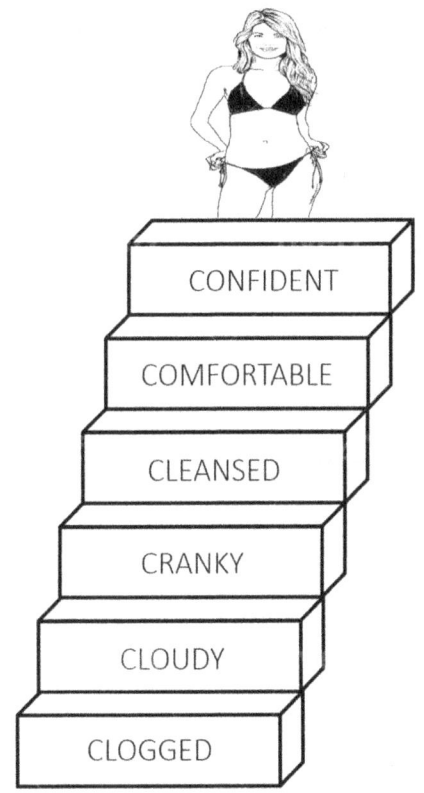

Aligned action - supporting bowel health

- **Cleanse your colon.** Check out https://balancedbabes.net/coloncleanse/ to download your free cleanse protocol including various cleanse options, eating plan, instructional videos and recommended supportive cleanse products.

- **Experiment with an enema.**
  Check out https://balancedbabes.net/enemas/
- **Eat more fruit and vegetables.** 10 serves of veggies and 3-5 serves of fruit daily.
- **Drink more water.** A minimum of 2 to 3 litres of filtered water daily. Start every morning by drinking one litre of water - it's only four glasses - and always have it done within the first hour of waking. Drinking warm water with lemon juice is an amazing way to stimulate your digestive system and get those bowels moving.
- **Consume more raw food.** Invest in a juicer. This is the best way to flood your body with the electricity of natural raw food which helps to stimulate bowel movements and smash out your 10 serves of veggies daily. Check out https://balancedbabes.net/resources/ for a list of affordable, good quality cold-pressed juicing machines.
- **Exercise.** Just 20 minutes of body movement is enough to stimulate your circulation and wake things up down thereby engaging your muscles and moving everything around in your body.
- **Abdominal massage.** Use a gentle carrier oil like almond or avocado with some essential oils like ginger, fennel, cardamom or fenugreek. Massage your tummy in a circular motion, starting on the right-hand side of your body, following the natural line of the colon. Doing this consistently over time will help to reengage the nerves within your digestive system and help with bloating.

Spiritual shape-up

Now, let's take a look at the spiritual and emotional meaning behind constipation. What it symbolises is not letting go.

Journaling the journey

- Where are you not letting go?
- What things in your life or what people in your life are you not letting go of?
- Where in your life are you full of shit and not living authentically?
- What grudges are you holding onto?
- Who do you need to forgive?
- What shame do you hold around poo and going to the toilet?
- What is your earliest memory surrounding toilet training and going to the toilet?

Get cracking with your self-awareness process. Listen to the 7 Step Hormone Healing guided meditation and explore these questions in your journal. Don't forget to ask your body questions and tune into the awareness and sensations that drop in.

*We recommend you read Chapters 6 and 7 consecutively and implement the recommendations at the same time as these protocols work hand in hand and are most effectively performed together.

CHAPTER 7

WHAT'S BUGGING YOU?

parasite
/ˈparəsʌɪt/

noun

an organism that lives in or on an organism of another species (its host) and benefits by deriving nutrients at the other's expense.

Unwanted, uninvited, parasites, bugs, harmful bacteria, viruses and infections! These suckers are undoubtedly the most underdiagnosed underlying contributor of hormonal imbalance and general disease from autoimmunity, cancers, depression, and everything in between regarding human health. The biggest issue is that they're largely unidentified; most of us don't even know we have these foreign invaders living inside us because when it comes to infections there's a huge difference between acute and chronic.

An acute infection is one that you know about; you feel like crap, it comes on suddenly presenting with a high temperature, hot sweats, headache, extreme fatigue and achy joints in response to your immune system swiftly responding to the 'emergency' change within your internal environment. A chronic infection, however, is one which lasts a long time, longer than three months, and is quite often asymptomatic. This becomes the taxing tug of war on your body as the immune system tries to fight what can only be described as a losing battle.

Here's the deal. If you've got a pathogen that is sneakily living rent-free in your body, it's going to mess up your hormones and slowly, steadily pollute your internal environment with its excrements and toxic waste products. Don't get me wrong, there's a big difference between good and bad foreign organisms, some pathogens can actually be beneficial for the human body, living symbiotically and improving your health. But when they start to overrun the joint, the friendship turns sour. These nasties can go largely unnoticed because the symptoms they create can be easily put down to everyday niggles and general poor lifestyle choices, like how you feel when you overeat, don't have enough sleep or just having an off day. Digestive discomfort, low energy, reoccurring acute infections (ear, urinary, chest), coughs, colds, aching joints, all quite mundane hardly serious stuff which doesn't exactly prompt you to investigate further, especially not without the high temp and severe pain of an 'acute' infection. And even if you did suspect a freeloader on board, quite often a routine stool test through your GP fails to detect evidence of these critters because their activity is always changing and we're not always actively excreting their remnants through our bowel motions. Blood tests can identify acute infections based on raised white blood cells and inflammatory markers but it's the low grade, long term chronic infections that we are completely unaware of that slowly sabotage our health and unbalance our hormones in the long run.

And here's why. If you are harbouring a low-grade infection or any organism that shouldn't be there, it's going to automatically put your body into a version of the flight and fight response we chatted about in Chapter 5. Your body is aware there's a foreign invader which activates the response, the immune system gets to work, the adrenal glands are alerted, and a stress response follows. However, these types of foreign invaders have evolved and adapted to a point they are now utilising their own inbuilt shields and biofilms, which makes it very difficult for the immune system to penetrate and completely eradicate. At best your white blood cell army will keep it at bay, but over time these toxic freeloaders take their toll on your system and with your 'stress' response alerted, until that infection is eradicated, your body will always be on alert.

Look at viruses for example. We've all heard it before, once you have the virus in your system it will never go away, it is opportunistic, lying dormant until your immune system is suppressed and your vitality low enough that it can gain momentum. That's when you'll feel the effects of an acute infection at play: aching joints, headache, fever, rashes and so on. And that's the problem, they're always there, working away behind the scenes, producing heavy metals and other toxic by-products, which severely burdens the liver. Their inhabitance creates stress in your body, which then has your defence team working tirelessly around the clock to keep it under control. This takes its toll on the body and over time makes it more difficult for your body to relax into the parasympathetic nervous system, the optimal state for rest, repair and recharge. The adrenal glands remain on high alert and produce more cortisol in order to keep motivating the soldiers (white blood cells) and while you're engaged in a battle, aka the fight or flight response, your reproductive hormones get zero love, because in that moment your body's primary goal is to keep you alive, which 'reproductive organs' are not required for.

With extended periods of this stress, irregular changes to your oestrogen and progesterone start to play out. Progesterone in particular is metabolised along the same pathway of the adrenal hormones and so if progesterone deficiency becomes a major issue when stress is high, this is a big reason why menstrual cycles can get out of whack.

Concerning re-occurring infections, the issue is not merely that the bug keeps coming back, it's more that the rude 'mo-fo' never left the building. This is quite often due to the overuse of antibiotic therapy, which works quickly to reduce the activity of the foreign invader - namely bacterial infections - enabling you to feel completely better, but the underlying infection is rarely completely destroyed and remains in your system waiting for the next opportunity you let your guard down with late nights, a few weeks in a row of poor eating, and then the infection reoccurs.

Urinary tract infections are a classic example of this and with the bug still lurking around your urinary canal each time a 'trigger' occurs, like sexual activity, not drinking enough water, consuming too much alcohol or not peeing often enough, this bug is able to breed up again and the signs of acute infection re-emerge. But this time the bug is stronger as it has already had a taste of the antibiotics in the past, so it knows how to arm itself, and your immune system is weaker due to the previous exposure to the immune-suppressing side effects of antibiotics.

The major culprit in reoccurring infections is the streptococcus infection, commonly identified by the medical system as Group A or B, although popular health professional Anthony William, the Medical Medium, believes there are far more variations of the strep family which are yet to be discovered, all playing equal havoc within our systems due to their excellent ability to adapt to antibiotic therapy. In fact, not only are antibiotics inadequate at treating strep infections, they actually feed and strengthen the infection and damage the liver in the process. Different strains are more aggressive than others but nonetheless this genius of bacterium is the culprit for many reoccurring infections such as ear, sinus, throat, respiratory infections, urinary tract and even acne.

Bacterial vaginosis a very common 'female' vaginal infection, also caused by this same strep family, but is quite often misdiagnosed as candida overgrowth. However, 'thrush' due to the overgrowth of the candida yeast, 99% of the time only occurs due to the underlying strep infection disabling our immune system, feeding the candida and with the addition of antibiotics strengthening this scenario, ineffective use of anti-fungal creams and capsules prescribed to counteract the discomfort of the candida overgrowth which only fuels the strep infection further. In this case the candida will never be managed if the cause of the overgrowth is not addressed, which stretches far beyond the over-consumption of sugars and yeast products.

Unfortunately, this is a cycle which quite often begins in babies when experiencing their first ear infection and due to the lack of understanding of the long term consequences of antibiotics, are given their first dose rather than treated safely and effectively with natural remedies, which is highly effective while the infection is quite controllable. Once the antibiotics are administered, the war begins, allowing strep to mutate into a monster that will continue to wreak havoc in your system for many years to come. Strep is often passed on by mum through childbirth; quite often ingested through animal proteins - meat, dairy, eggs which have been exposed to antibiotics or genetically through generations of antibiotic abuse. Even if a child was not directly exposed to antibiotics, strep is still a very real problem for many, especially regarding acne.

Hormonal or cystic acne is a classic example of 'shooting the messenger' but the truth is, your acne has nothing to do with your hormones and everything to do with the underlying strep infection which is weakening your liver, immune and lymphatic systems.

The hormonal changes which occur at puberty around ovulation and the menstrual bleed, temporarily suppress the immune system as the body prioritises more energy and attention on your reproductive cycle, which results in the reduced productivity of the white blood cells. This allows the once-contained strep infection (thanks to your liver) to now escape and enter the lymphatic system as it sets off for the subcutaneous fat layer under your skin where it feeds and breeds.

Unfortunately, this layer of fat is also a major source of toxins, stored antibiotics and anti-fungal drugs which the body hasn't been able to fully metabolise and excrete over the years, allowing the strep to multiply. Naturally your trusty immune system rushes to the scene of the crime in an attempt to contain the infection, resulting in pussy spots (clumps of white blood cells) or at the very least raised red lumps from the inflammation and accumulation of white blood cells as the war in your skin unfolds.

Quite often women observe the correlation between consuming dairy and skin breakouts because it is this mucus-forming source of animal fat which creates the sluggishness in the lymphatic system, making it harder for white blood cells to identify and attack the strep. The same applies to wheat, which strep also loves to feed on.

Now don't get me wrong, antibiotics have their place, especially concerning life-threatening infections, but they've been abused and over-prescribed in non-life-threatening situations, allowing these organisms to adapt, creating superbugs completely resistant to antibiotics.

Through my years of working with chronic, hormone-related reproductive disorders from endometriosis, libido issues, fibromyalgia, auto-immune conditions, PMS, adrenal fatigue, thyroid imbalances, cystic ovaries, infertility and so on, there is always the presence of a chronic underlying infection, affecting the body's ability to heal and maintain balance. And until the infection is completely eradicated and your body is able to get off the 'flight or fight' merry-go-round, you will never move forward with your healing journey. Addressing this issue is non-negotiable and must be done in conjunction with cleansing the colon as part of a holistic approach, which addresses the conjunctive causative factors contributing to the disease state. In this case, the excessive congestion and build-up of mucoid plaque within the colon acts as a hospitable breeding environment for the pathogens, allowing them to flourish and continue to gain momentum.

Another classic example of foreign invaders affecting reproductive health is undiagnosed infections occurring within the uterus. This is quite often the cause of failed IVF attempts and early miscarriages, by which these low-grade chronic infections mess with the normal healthy flora of the uterus. It is at this stage of infection, when the body is quite often losing the fight that natural killer cells are activated, a cytotoxic lymphocyte which produces chemicals to destroy tumours and infected tissue. The problem is, when these cells build up in the womb due to the infection, when pregnancy occurs, the developing foetus is very much caught in the crossfire of the natural immune response, resulting in miscarriage. This is a similar phenomenon which occurs in all auto-immune related conditions. It is naïve to conclude that the immune system simply turns on itself and begins to attack your own body; there is a sequence of events which take place creating the inflammatory response but ultimately your immune system is merely trying to attack the foreign invader living within your tissue, making it a messy battlefield.

Attempts to suppress your immune system with immune-suppressant drugs or anti-coagulant therapy will always fall short without first addressing the reason why your immune system is behaving the way it is. When it comes to health, it is important to understand the innate intelligence of our body and its ability to heal itself. Nothing ever occurs without reason and if we can look beyond the surface of symptoms and truly explore why the body is doing what it is doing, only then can we achieve optimal health. Humans mistakenly thinking they know better than mother nature and the creation of the human body has ultimately lead to their own demise, creating chronic illness.

How do I know if I have a chronic infection?

The reality is, we're exposed to many pathogens on a daily basis, through the air, our water supply, walking barefoot on the ground, exposure to others with infections, consuming raw meats and eggs, eating food that's been left out too long, poor hygiene practices, stagnant water, insect bites and many more. The real question is, how is it possible you DON'T have an underlying invader stressing your system! But this is not about throwing our hands in the air and continuing to bury our head in the sand. Your best defence against these critters is ensuring your immune system is strong and healthy.

So, how do you work out whether or not you actually have an infection? Especially if you've seen your GP and there are no abnormalities in your blood screening, and a stool sample also came back clear. When it comes to making this self-assessment, you need to look at the whole picture including your health history and start to listen to the clues your body is giving you. What are the symptoms you are experiencing on a day-to-day basis? Are you trying different things but still not seeing any improvement with your health and wellbeing? Do your symptoms change from day to day? Do you react to certain foods one day but not the next? When it feels like your health is starting to get more and more 'out of your control', despite all your best efforts to seek help, change your diet and support your body, quite often, your health is out of your control when you are at the mercy of a foreign invader or infection.

If testing is an avenue you are adamant about exploring, a comprehensive stool analysis through a functional medicine practitioner or natural therapist is a great way to thoroughly investigate what's actually depleting your body and vitality. These tests are a substantial investment, but well worth the money if you've been suffering from debilitating health issues for an extended period of time, especially auto-immune conditions. Taking a holistic approach to your gut health by identifying the health of your microbiome through these comprehensive investigations which look at bacteriology culture identifying and differentiating between the various forms of beneficial bacteria and dysbiotic flora, yeast cultures, parasitology, digestion and absorption markers, inflammation, immunology, short-chain fatty acids and intestinal health markers is life-changing for someone with chronic disease. On average I find that those suffering from chronic illness have five different strains of harmful resistant bacteria in their bodies that are preventing them from healing, but once these infections are eradicated, health begins to thrive.

Signs you have a chronic infection:

- Aching joints
- Acne
- Allergies
- Brain fog
- Chronic conditions such as auto-immune conditions, endometriosis, chronic fatigue syndrome
- Headaches
- Low energy
- Low mood
- Recurrent infections: UTI's, chronic candida infections
- SIBO – small intestinal bacterial overgrowth
- Thick greenish coating on the base of the tongue
- Ongoing digestive problems
- Unrefreshed sleep.

Fighting mystery infections certainly isn't an easy overnight quest. It takes time, consistent application and a holistic, safe approach which more often than not results in you feeling worse in the short term, before your health takes a positive step in the right direction. Treating the body holistically is undoubtedly 'hard work' because it's actually stopping and listening to what your body requires and addressing each individual disconnect, imbalance, deficiency, toxicity and linking everything together whilst supporting the system and considering the long term consequences of your treatment approach and what effect it has on overall health.

Ignoring the underlying infection in your body which is slowly but surely depleting your immune system, taxing your adrenal and nervous systems, polluting your body and burdening your liver is kinda like refusing to acknowledge the white elephant in the room. It will not go away on its own. Your body is incredible, and it is equipped with the tools and ability to heal itself, but due to the overuse of 'scientifically sound' medical and pharmaceutical interventions, environmental pollutions, the development of electromagnetic frequencies, radiation, the depletion of minerals in our soils and so forth, our bodies are now under more strain than ever and staying healthy now requires a more concentrated effort than ever before.

Health is your birthright, but it is also your responsibility. It's your job to practice a level of self-awareness every single day by acknowledging how the foods, thoughts, environments and people we surround ourselves with have an effect on our health. It's our job to question everything, how it specifically affects your individual system, especially the scientifically backed practices. Living under the premise that 'it will not happen to me' or 'I'll deal with it once I'm sick' is now resulting in more and more people coming undone with more chronic illness in society than ever before. Alzheimer's disease, diabetes, heart disease, cancer, none of these things happen by accident, they are all the result of long-term stress, depletion and imbalance within the body that the host failed to recognise or failed to act upon soon enough.

Treating infections

Treating your infections is a 3-part process, which must be done specifically in this order to completely eradicate the infection, and to support your body through the 'war' in the process.

There are many natural 'anti-microbial' herbs, vitamins, minerals, foods and essential oils which have a powerful action on destroying and disarming pathogens within your body. Natural, typically means they are derived from nature or of a non-chemical nature which means they are less harsh on your system and don't add to the toxic burden in your body as many pharmaceutical anti-viral, antibiotics, anti-fungal solutions. We must not underestimate that these agents still need to be treated with caution and must be used correctly. We must also understand that due to the rapid adaptation of viruses, parasites, bacteria, fungi, yeast and other harmful organism it's important to administer these agents in a way that will not do more harm than good and support the eradication process concomitantly.

Acute infections

If you had to lift 1000 heavy bricks from one end of the yard to the other, even if you knew you could physically do it all on your own, but it would take a lot longer, would you appreciate an extra few pairs of hands to help you do the job? This is exactly how it is when your body gets sick with a cold. You have an immune system which is designed to get in and fight that cold, but if you can help your immune system do the job by supporting it with natural, scientifically proven, therapeutic immune boosters and anti-microbial support, your body appreciates the helping hand.

Here's what to do when you get struck with an acute infection – be it the common cold, mastitis, a swollen gland, an infected cut or cellulitis. If you can, load your body with supportive nutrition to stimulate the production of white blood cells, to recruit a stronger army to override the infection more quickly. You will recover faster but you'll also ensure your immune system isn't completely wiped out, making you more susceptible to infection down the track and you'll have a much better chance of completely eradicating the infection in its entirety.

- **Eat raw garlic.** Always crush the garlic to activate the active constituent, mix it with some manuka or raw honey and take several times a day. Just don't do it on an empty stomach, it burns, and yes, you will have the smell of garlic coming out your pores for a couple of days, but this is a highly effective method which is just as effective as antibiotic therapy, especially for resistant chest infections.
- **Drink fresh lemon juice and raw or manuka honey**
- **Eat loads of citrus fruits high in Vitamin C as well as kiwi fruit, strawberries and pineapple**
- **Supplement with a combination of one of the following natural anti-viral, anti-bacterial, immune-boosting agents:** Andrographis, Colloidal silver, Elderberry, Echinacea, Goldenseal, Medicinal Mushrooms, Olive leaf, Vitamin C, Zinc.
- **Drink loads of water**

- **Rest**: use your sick leave. You're sick because your body wants a reset, so slow down and allow the body to fight the battle, then recover.

Chronic infections

Dealing with chronic infections is a much more complex process due to the long-standing invasion which has enabled the organism to build in numbers and adapt itself to anti-microbial agents, be they natural or pharmaceutical. The following principles therefore must be applied.

1. Treat or attack the infection consistently over an extended period of time.
2. Choose a dose of your anti-microbial which is potent enough to have an effect on the body but doesn't burden your own system too much.
3. Choose a specific remedy which has a broad spectrum of anti-microbial activity with a specific affinity to the suspected nature of your infection. Viral, bacterial, fungal, parasite etc.

My recommendation for working with resistant infections is to attack from all angles, a process I refer to as 'bug blasting'. Don't get me wrong, this is a heavy-duty plan of attack and must be done responsibly or you can deplete your gut microbiome, vitality and resistance.

Bug blasting

Stage 1

- **Heavy-duty, broad-spectrum anti-microbial therapy.** This includes anti-viral herbs as well as a potent anti-microbial agent known as grapeseed extract. Now, this is a controversial approach. Although completely natural, grapeseed is very powerful in its activity, with the fear among many practitioners that it is too powerful and completely destroys the natural GIT microbiome in the process, which is no different to antibiotics.

And although I agree, I still believe grapeseed extract is a superior choice for long-standing resistant infections because it does not contain the toxic residue that pharmaceuticals create and if prescribed appropriately with supportive probiotic therapy and immune stimulants, we can prevent the damage to your microbiome. But you MUST support the process and protect your gut microbiome with the below processes. Alternatively, other effective natural anti-microbials which can be used include:

- Oregano
- Thyme
- Garlic
- Uva ursi
- Caprylic acid
- Berberine
- Rosemary
- Sage
- Basil
- Cardamom
- Clove

- **Disarm the shield** - Biofilms are tiny communities of cells that grow on surfaces or organisms. They are difficult to penetrate and have been found to be involved in the following disease states:
    - Arterial plaque
    - Chronic sinus infections
    - Chronic wounds
    - Cystic fibrosis
    - Inner ear infections
    - Kidney stones
    - Osteonecrosis
    - Periodontal disease
    - Urinary tract infections
    - Lyme disease

Addressing the biofilm can be done with therapeutic products such as proteolytic enzymes, n-acetyl cysteine and essential oils such as:

- Peppermint essential oil
- Thyme essential oil
- Tea tree oil
- **Supplement the gastro-intestinal microflora** – bug blasting includes the use of multi-anti-microbial therapy which over an extended period of time will have a detrimental effect on your healthy bacteria, which is why the bug blasting is done in a cyclical nature and always supported with rest and restoration periods. Use supportive probiotics **because** the anti-microbial agent you use will destroy some of the beneficial bacteria in your system as well. It's highly important to use a concurrent broad-spectrum multi-strain probiotic at the same time. Simply dose this at least two hours away from your anti-microbial.
- **Support the liver** - The 'die-off' effect can be quite harsh on the liver and your system in general, so helping the liver with supportive herbs to prevent classic die-off symptoms such as headaches, fatigue and skin breakouts is necessary.
- **Cycle it on and off** - Never use anti-microbials for an extended period of time; sometimes 7-21 days at a time with a 7-14 day break minimum, then repeating the process until the infection is eradicated. This allows your immune system to stay strong, protects your natural gut microbiome and also helps your liver stay on top of the process.

Stage 2 - Supportive therapy and microbiome building through the break periods

Yes, absolutely fighting infections can be done incorrectly and cause issues if we go at it like a bull at a gate. It's super important to protect your natural gastrointestinal flora, the healthy bugs, and not wipe these out in the process, which involves taking into consideration the duration of your treatment blocks and the rest periods by which we focus purely of replenishing and recovering the gut. To soothe and support the gut lining it's important to use stuff like slippery elm powder, glutamine, aloe vera juice, chamomile tea, turmeric and a broad-spectrum probiotic formula.

When we start the war and start to attack these nasty invaders, the body experiences something called the 'die-off effect' which results in the excretion of toxic by-products and the putrefaction of the dying organisms, which has a harmful effect on the liver, which has to mop up the mess.

Stage 3 – Build the immune system

Build a stronger army! Your white blood cells play a huge supporting role in this protocol, especially in the clean-up process. The macrophage, a large white blood cell, has the job of locating foreign bodies, including toxins, cell debris, organisms and engulfing them. Think of these guys as the rubbish disposal guys who come along and clean up the battlefield. When you've been dealing with an infestation of any unwanted microbial in your body for an extended period of time, it's a taxing process on the body and it's really important to keep your immune system boosted as you can be more susceptible to picking up additional acute infections like colds, while on the protocol.

Using immune-boosting foods like:

- Citrus fruits, including the peel and pips in juices
- Pineapple
- Raw honey
- Garlic
- Ginger
- Blueberries
- Turmeric
- Sweet potato
- Pumpkin
- Onions
- Carrots
- Parsnips
- Shiitake mushrooms
- Cayenne pepper
- Oregano
- Rosemary

You can also use herbs and nutrients which double by supporting the adrenal glands and helps to build your immune system whilst replenishing the overworked, overstressed adrenal glands.

- Olive leaf
- Turmeric
- Echinacea
- Zinc
- Vitamin C
- Astragalus
- Licorice
- Siberian ginseng

Sunshine

There's so much fear around the sun and exposing ourselves to sunshine these days, but the reality is, sunlight will help to support your immune system by boosting vitamin D levels. Deficiency in vitamin D is associated with increased autoimmunity as well as increased susceptibility to infection, so getting a regular dose of sunshine is important. Just do it wisely; stay out of the hottest periods of the day between 10am and 2pm when the UV rays are at their most intense. Your body uses vitamins and minerals to protect itself from UV damage, so the more nutritionally depleted you are, the more easily you'll burn in the sun.

Make a cold-pressed juice your daily medicine. Not only can you get a hit of at least five vegetables in one go, this superfood cocktail is far more beneficial to your body than any synthetically produced multi-vitamin that you'll more than likely struggle to absorb. There's really no comparison between lab-produced vitamins vs naturally occurring vitamins in freshly grown food. They are worlds apart. Let's just say, although synthetically produced vitamins have their place and can definitely have a therapeutic effect on the body, they should be considered medicine, not nutrition. Natural vitamins and minerals are like the key which unlocks the door to health and the synthetic counterpart is kinda like a heavyweight which just tries to bang the door down with force; completely ignorant to any destruction it's causing in the process.

As an extra immune boost, never underestimate the power of exercise in stimulating the immune and lymphatic systems, by increasing the circulation and flow of lymph fluid, which contains white blood cells, creating a more effective 'clean up' fighting off infections and removing foreign debris. When we remain sedentary our body does too. No movement = no life. Infrared saunas and drinking herbal teas such as echinacea, elderberry, orange and cinnamon are another great way to keep your immune system firing!

Boost your immune system with natural immunity, by being happy, enjoying lots of sunshine, drinking lots of water, and making sure you're nutritionally sound. This means not depleting any of your major 'things,' especially vitamin C and zinc, vitamin E, vitamin A, and all those other amazing immune-boosting vitamins.

Remember – not everyone has the vitality to withstand bug blasting. Your adrenal health and immunity is the first checkpoint. If you identify with adrenal exhaustion and your immune system is already struggling based on frequent colds and acute infections, you must first build your immune system up with an immune-boosting protocol and work consistently on your adrenal health before undertaking bug blasting.

Step 3 - Recovering from Resistant Infections

Diagram: Circular diagram with central hexagon labeled "Infected & Irritated to Invincible Immunity" surrounded by six segments: ANTI-MICROBIAL TREATMENT, BIOFILM BREAK DOWN, SUPPORT THE LIVER, RESTORE GUT MICROBIOME, CLEAR COLON CONGESTION, HEAL THE GUT.

Case study

Michael, age 52 presented with excessive fatigue, weight gain that would not budge, aching joints, chronic digestive disturbances including pain, bloating, gas, distention, insane brain fog and was picking up regular acute infections due to the suppressed state of his immune system.

A comprehensive stool analysis on 8/7/2018 revealed the following imbalanced flora, aka 'bad bacteria' in his system:
- 4+ Bifidobacterium spp.
- 2+ Alpha hemolytic strep
- 1+ Beta strep, group B
- 4+ Gamma hemolytic strep

2+ Klebsiella pneumoniae ssp pneumoniae
2+ Lactococcus lactis
2+ Providencia alcalifaciens

Additionally, he had an overgrowth of clostridium spp., which is harmful when present in high quantities, as well as zero growth of Lactobacillus, a beneficial bacterium. Michael also had moderate amounts of the parasite blastocystis hominis and large amounts of candida albicans which had multiplied out of control due to the underlying resistant infections.

After three rounds of the above treatment protocol which included supplementation with grapeseed extract for 14-21 days followed by a rest period of 7-14 days using a gut healing probiotic powder cycled on and off, additional herbal liver support, n-acetyl cysteine to disarm the biofilm on the 22/10/2018, all seven of the infections had been eradicated and all of his symptoms subsided, including clear thinking, improved memory and concentration, healthy, happy digestive system, no pain, and the weight around his mid-centre was now starting to shift.

What's more, after the three cycles of the aggressive 'bug blasting,' his beneficial bacteria remained healthy and strong enough to maintain digestive health and immunity.

Beneficial bacteria before commencing therapy

4+ Bacteroides fragilis group
4+ Bifidobacterium spp.
2+ Escherichia coli
NG Lactobacillus spp.
1+ Enterococcus spp.
4+ Clostridium spp.

Beneficial Bacteria after commencing therapy

    3+ Bacteroides fragilis group
    3+ Bifidobacterium spp.
    3+ Escherichia coli
    2+ Lactobacillus spp.
    3+ Enterococcus spp.
    3+ Clostridium spp.

Key – NG: No Growth, 1+ less than 1,000 CFUs/gm, 2+ 1,000 – 10,000 CFUs/gm, 3+ 100,000 – 1,000,000 CFUs/gm 4+ More than 10,000,000 CFUs/gm

CFUs = Colony-forming units = Single viable organisms/per gram of stool tested

For more information on how to treat underlying, recurrent infections in your body, checkout out the Balanced Babes treatment protocols https://balancedbabes.net/treatmentprotocols/

Spiritual shape-up

In your chilled out space, grab your journal, do the meditation, and then ask yourself the following questions.

Journaling the Journey

- **What's bugging you?**
- **What is sucking the life out of you?**
- **Where are you giving away your power?**
- **Who is the parasite in your life?**

CHAPTER 8

THIS GIRL IS ON FIRE

"We're all born with livers that are already weakened, toxins are passed down the family line, we inherit them at conception and in the womb. And then our livers are barraged by a wide range of toxins throughout the entire course of our lives because of the imperfect modern world we live in."

Anthony William, The Medical Medium

Have you ever felt so angry you felt out of control? The rage so big it feels like your blood is literally boiling? Well, from a traditional Chinese medicine perspective, this is exactly what happens when the liver is angry! Our livers are completely overwhelmed by their job to detoxify and eliminate toxic chemicals and then on top of that bombarded with negative emotions such as fear and anxiety. This leads to the production of stress chemicals that the liver has to deal with, that it literally can set the liver on fire due to the heat that this process creates in the body.

'Liver fire' is a common phenomenon causing suffering among many, but which came first, the rage or the heat? Actually, it's a two-way street. The heat is the consequence of poorly managed stress and reactive behaviour as well as the stress of ageing and toxic overload in the body. Heat in the liver creates anger and anger creates heat in the liver! This affects the flow of energy, aka the 'qi' through the body resulting in stagnation of the blood and 'fire' which weakens the liver even further and the cycle continues.

If you're someone who struggles with excessive heat and a 'cranky' liver, you'll recognise the symptoms all too well: a dry mouth, eyes and throat, red eyes and face, irritability, outbursts of anger, dizziness, ringing in the ears, excessive thirst, bitter taste in the mouth, muscle tightness in the neck and shoulders, migraines and headaches, especially on the sides of the head, a general feeling of 'warmth', blood pressure issues, dark urine, insomnia and our good old friend constipation.

A stressed-out liver is very much a contributing factor in the complex puzzle of 'healthy hormone balance' and one that cannot be ignored! Welcome to Step 4, loving your liver!

Your poor old liver is the most loyal organ you have, hardworking, modest, forgiving and never expecting any spotlight, despite the fact it's saving your life every day. Without it you'd more or less die a quick and painful death, drowning in your own toxic filth, which is why this organ is one of the top five vital organs of the human body, yet probably the most ignored.

The liver works tirelessly all day, every day, keeping your body clean. Filtering the toxins we're exposed to in this toxic world we inhabit. The toxins we inhale from environmental pollutions, industrial chemicals, building materials, the chemicals in the fabrics of the clothing we wear, our toxic beauty care regime and the endocrine disruptors we unknowingly put on our skin, the processed foods we eat that our bodies don't like, pesticides, herbicides, alcohol, pharmaceutical drugs, refined sugars, cleaning products, toxic printing materials on transaction receipts, plastics and printing materials.

But it doesn't stop there. Those pesky foreign invaders we chatted about in the last chapter secreting their excrements and heavy metals, the generational stuff that's been passed down from mum and dad that we ever so kindly inherit at the time of conception as our genetic blueprint is formed. It doesn't seem to matter where you look, we're surrounded by toxins all day, every day. Sadly, this is just another 'effect' of the industrial revolution, advances in technology and the modern-day conveniences we are privileged to enjoy, and prefer to keep in our lives, which of course is okay. But let's start to acknowledge it and stop living in denial. When we know better, we can do better and start to make more educated, informed decisions about the things we choose to expose ourselves to and actions to protect our bodies and help our liver!

I'm not suggesting that we all need to throw all our plastics in the bin, stop wearing make-up, burn down our houses and go and live in the wilderness. Obviously, that's not practical; I for one happen to love the comfort of my new age lifestyle and all that we have access to, but I'm aware of the effect it's having on my body and I choose to implement practices to counteract how it affects my health in the long run.

We do, however, need to be willing to implement changes to our life which must begin with recognising and respecting the liver and all it does for us, which is probably a whole lot more than you realise. The liver stores vitamins and minerals to prepare for times of need. It regulates and stores glucose and glycogen for healthy blood sugar levels and energy utilisation. It processes fats and helps you maintain your ideal weight. It detoxifies dangerous heavy metals and it even supports your immune system by fighting infections with its own innate immune processes. And the most important thing to note is the involvement our liver has on our hormones. You will never maintain happy, healthy balanced hormones if your liver is overworked and underpaid. Along with all the other lifesaving tricks your body has in place, the liver will also prioritise keeping you alive above anything else, so unfortunately addressing critical changes in blood sugar levels, detonating heavy metal bombs and containing dangerous infections from the systemic circulation will always trump your reproductive hormones, leaving them vulnerable to neglect in a stressed-out body!

Remember, your worn-out adrenal system which utilises the 'fight or flight' mechanism to keep your body from danger, well that also impacts your liver health. When we're stressed out and living in that hyper-stimulated 'fight or flight' state, producing high amounts of adrenaline and cortisol, the liver has to clean up the aftermath. So, girlfriend if you're always on edge, your liver has a full-time job processing your stress chemicals alone. You are probably starting to realise pretty quickly that your body, without particularly trying, has become a dirty minefield of toxins! And while we're on that subject, just to clarify, a toxin is a poisonous substance produced within living cells, organisms or synthetically produced by artificial processes and when the liver can't keep up with the clean-up, your body really starts to feel the effects of this toxic burden. Think:

- Dark circles under the eyes
- Skin breakouts
- Low energy
- Digestive disturbances
- Headaches
- Feeling heavy bloated and congested
- Brown spots on the skin.

These are a few signs your liver isn't keeping up with the workload. What your body is really trying to tell you with those 'annoying, inconvenient symptoms' is, "hey I need a bit of help here, I'm struggling to detoxify and eliminate these dangerous chemicals from your precious body and now they're starting to hurt you". This is your body communicating that your liver is overworked, and you need to make some simple lifestyle changes to help minimise your exposure to these daily chemicals, and what it would really love is a break. A detox.

Now, I know the 'D' word is a dirty one for most. The thought of restricting yourself from the convenience and joy of your daily indulgences and going without coffee and chocolate sends a shiver down most people's spines! We imagine it as a prison sentence, not being able to eat anything, go anywhere or do anything all the while feeling like death. But just like cleaning your fish tank it's one of those things no one really likes to do but is highly necessary in order to sustain the health, happiness and wellbeing of your beloved pet. Do you see where I'm going with this? Internal body cleansing is just as important as washing your external body.

Do I really need to detox?

Detoxing or cleansing, whichever sounds less scary to you, is very much about loving yourself enough to give your body a spring clean to ensure your health and longevity prevails. Loving the liver and helping it out from time to time is the one thing you are going to wish you had prioritised annually when you are deep in your suffering with chronic disease or facing a cancer diagnosis. When the body is toxic it affects the normal functioning of ALL of your systems, including your immune system, circulatory system, lymphatic system and nervous system. No cell in your body is safe if it's drowning in toxic waste. I cannot stress highly enough the role in cleansing your body of toxicity in disease prevention and health promotion. It is simply non-negotiable.

There will be some of you reading this who feel this doesn't apply, because perhaps you're one of the lucky ones with a strong constitution who rarely gets sick and feels like your health is pretty good. You don't get headaches, your skin is flawless and you're having no issues with your weight (lucky you), and in this situation, it would be super easy to overlook the importance of cleansing. However, naively thinking your liver is fine because your latest blood tests said so is one of the biggest mistakes you can make. I hate sounding all dramatic and sinister, but sister, EVERYONE's liver is struggling, yours included, whether you feel it yet or not. The level of toxicity in our environment is far greater than our body can keep up with and eventually the balance will be turned if you're not taking targeted action to protect and support your natural detoxification processes. Toxicity will eventually catch up.

Daily detox

Never underestimate the 1%'ers. Every single action you do or don't do on a daily basis is contributing to your health. Just for a moment think of your health like a bank account. Let's just say when you were born, you were given a million dollars to open your account. And each time you encounter something which negatively affects your health, like inhaling a puff of cigarette smoke, eating a deep-fried rancid fat engorged potato chip or injecting yourself with a heavy metal filled vaccine, you lose a dollar or two. But for every cold-pressed vegetable juice, session of exercise or burst of serotonin after a connecting with loved ones, you're able to replenish the bank account. All you've got to do is ensure you're earning as much as your spending, right? This is where the daily detox principles come in. These are long term gentle 'money earners' for your health which help your liver stay on top of its game keeping up with the toxic burden, which is damaging your cells, rapidly ageing you and robbing you of vitality. These are things which have a gentle effect on the body and can be safely done by all ages, all sexes and even pregnant or breast-feeding mama's and these are the things your liver truly appreciates.

Enemas: This is an amazing way to 'express' the release of stagnant toxins within your colon and exit them quick smart from your body.

Plants inside your home: Not only do they look delightful in the home, they actually protect you from electro-magnetic frequencies from Wi-Fi which can help to improve your energy levels and reduce the level of stress on your physical body.

Infrared saunas: Through the process of sweating we are able to accelerate the elimination of toxins through the skin. Infrared saunas are believed to be more effective than traditional saunas because it allows for the removal of not just water through sweat, but also cholesterol, fat-soluble toxins, toxic heavy metals, sulfuric acid, sodium, ammonia and uric acid.

Drinking cold-pressed juice daily: The influx of easy to absorb and digest nutrients from fresh fruit and vegetables floods the body with vitamins, minerals and antioxidants which are vital ingredients in the phase 1, 2 and 3 liver detoxification pathways by which harmful chemicals are converted into water-soluble molecules which can be safely eliminated from the body.

Move your bowels 2-3 times daily: As your major elimination channel, it's vital that your bowels open regularly to prevent the reabsorption of chemicals back into your system through the semi-permeable membrane that is your bowel wall.

Fresh air: Eliminate toxic air fresheners and sprays from your home. Breathing in these chemicals overloads your liver just as quickly as consuming chemicals in your diet. Make an effort to spend a portion of your day outside in circulating fresh air. Your lungs, another key elimination organ also loves this!

Eat organic: Sure, it's not always possible to do this 100% of the time, but where you can, choose organic which hasn't been doused in chemical sprays and even better start growing your own herbs and fresh veggies. No matter your space, there's always a way with innovative new growing ideas available on the internet.

Clean up your beauty regime: Check out the list of ingredients in your makeup and hair and skincare products. 90% of these are of chemical origin and if it's being applied to your skin, it is ending up in your body. Switch your products to plant-based, organic natural alternatives.

Do a colon cleanse 1-4 times per year: This is kinda like emptying the bag of your vacuum cleaner and enjoying the benefits of the better performance after the cleanout.

Limit your exposure to chemicals in the home: The biggest source of chemicals is our cleaning products, but this can be easily substituted for natural organic options and even DIY homemade essential oil-based products which anyone can master with a little help from Google!

Get a water filter: This may be a bigger investment but considering your body requires 2-3 litres minimum a day to function optionally, you sure as hell want to make sure that 2-3 litres isn't laden with fluoride, chlorine, aluminium and all the other nasty bacterium and heavy metals found in your tank or the local water supply.

Take Epson (magnesium sulphate) salt baths: Soak your entire body in one cup of Epson salts if you have the luxury of a bathtub in your home, otherwise simply place your feet in a bucket large enough with the same amount of Epson salts. The body will rapidly absorb the salts which will not only support your magnesium levels and relax the muscles, but through the process of osmosis the minerals in the water are able to draw out impurities from the body.

Overwhelmed people do nothing, so start slowly and gradually experiment with all of the above recommendations. You don't need to implement all of these at once but give yourself the gift of good health by working these principles into your daily routine over time. Slow and steady wins the race of longevity! Make the time to research your options on the internet, join discussion groups on social media and prioritise putting away money to invest in the necessary items to allow these regimes to be effortless and consistent in your life.

Our Toxic Beauty Industry

Something that breaks my heart is the lack of regulation within the beauty industry. As women we often like to explore our creative feminine energy with makeup, colour and aromatising scents, but unfortunately this has become a toxic daily practice which is crippling our hormone health. The problem with this toxic industry is that there's very little awareness around the consequences of plastering our body with chemical ingredients on a daily basis and the long-term health effects. By law, cosmetic companies don't have to list certain ingredients and are entitled to claim their product is organic as long as it contains 80% organic ingredients, despite containing other dangerous non-organic ingredients.

Your skin is the largest organ in the human body and like your bowel wall, it's permeable, so anything that goes on your skin, ends up in your body.

The average woman uses between 5 and 20 products before even leaving the house of a morning - how many are you using? It's not that your toothpaste, shampoo, conditioner, blush, mascara, moisturiser, shaving gel, deodorant, lip gloss, concealer, hair spray or perfume are 'deadly' right then and there, but imagine the compounding effect as these daily products are used consistently every day. Your liver has to try and detoxify these chemicals, including endocrine disruptors on top of everything else it's exposed to and it's not an easy job. It's not your fault because until recent years there really hasn't been a lot of awareness surrounding the graveness of this issue, but with greater awareness, it is now your responsibility to choose what you put on your body.

The number one product I want you to start with is your aluminium-based deodorant. Aluminium is a known carcinogen linked with breast cancer and Alzheimer's disease and when applied directly to your armpit, a region concentrated with lymphatic tissue, directly linking to the breast tissue, it's a recipe for disaster overloading this nasty toxic heavy metal in such a delicate area with reduced circulation. Team this with underwire bras, which further reduce the blood flow and we have a stagnant area pooling in chemicals which over time damages the cells and weakens the immune system.

Here's the thing, when you change your deodorant to a natural non-toxic alternative, there's a fair chance you're going to stink in the beginning! When you stop clogging up your sweat glands with toxic antiperspirants your body will do what it is naturally designed to do; detoxify the dangerous chemicals. Releasing toxins directly through your sweat is going to produce a body odour. Short term stench is inevitable, so please persevere because you are doing one of the best cancer preventative measures you can by allowing your breast tissue to detoxify. You might like to make yourself a bentonite clay armpit mask to quicken the process. Drinking green juices including kale, spinach, alfalfa, lettuce and parsley loaded with natural chlorophyll is also a great way to naturally deodorise the smell of your body.

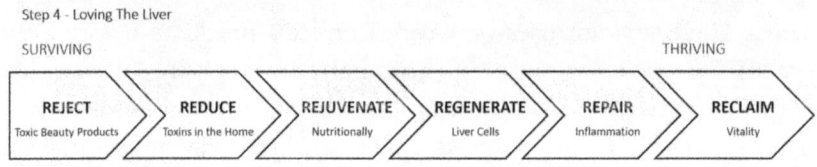

Concentrated cleansing - the Balanced Babes Babe cleanse

Introducing the Babe cleanse. I'm not going to lie to you, detoxing isn't necessarily always fun or easy, but since we're fast establishing it's a necessity for good health, you are going to want to have a regime you can implement year in and year out that is as painless as possible. Detoxification can make you feel pretty crappy, especially if it's not done safely, because the primary act of converting a toxin into something less dangerous takes its toll on the body and needs to be supported by the correct detoxification nutrients. Tiredness, headaches, aching muscles, insomnia, changes to your bowels, skin breakouts and body door are classic detox reactions and the common effect of moving toxins out of your body at a faster rate than normal as you start a detoxification program.

There's a lot of hype in social media in particular and companies trying to capitalise on the financial benefits of flogging off shoddy quick-fix detox and cleanse programs, but we must remember there is absolutely a chance of doing more harm than good if you do not adequately support yourself through a cleanse. There's also B grade programs which claim to cleanse yet still advocate the consumption of meat and animal products, which completely defies the traditional meaning of detoxification, as your liver will not get the 'rest and restoration' it requires through the process if it is still having to break down dense, acidic complex animal proteins. A true cleanse program will be 100% plant-based and may or may not include fasting, but it must include copious amounts of raw real food nutrition to really flush the liver and revive your toxic body.

Absolutely detoxing requires planning, preparation and supportive nutritional and herbal therapy to offset the side effects of detoxification. Although it's common to feel flat and headachy in the early days as your body withdraws from caffeine and sugar, if these symptoms persist there's a fair chance you are doing more harm than good, and your body is lacking the necessary supportive nutritional co-factors it requires to safely eliminate toxins. Think of vitamins and minerals as the bouncer which escorts unruly toxins out of the building. These toxins will not leave on their own accord and your body really does require that extra support to move them out, which is why juice fasting is a popular practice while detoxing due to the large amount of nutritional support they provide. Juice fasting really isn't for everyone though, especially if you are already adrenally depleted. Your first cleanse may just include going plant-based for a period of time and starting off more slowly whilst cleansing your colon and giving that liver a well-deserved holiday.

Detoxification really is an intricate process that has many elements which need to be considered in order to do it safely, which is why I designed the Balanced Babes Babe cleanse. The Babe cleanse includes everything you need to know about safe, effective cleansing, how to do it, when to do it, why to do it and how to support your body through the process. You can check this out at https://balancedbabes.net/babecleanse

Spiritual shape-up - unaddressed anger

So, as always, get in the habit of practising your daily meditation and tune in, go within, connect with your body, and ask your liver. Place your hands over your liver, which is on the right side of your body, below your rib cage and speak to it.

Journaling the Journey

- **How are you feeling?**
- **Are you struggling?**
- **What rage are you holding onto?**
- **Why are you angry?**
- **What are you angry at?**

CHAPTER 9

YOUR GUT IS YOUR GURU

"Your intestinal lining is about the size of a tennis court. Over 300 square meters in size, that's a lot of territory for beneficial bacteria to patrol and support health."

Dr Mercola

We're now living in an era where we're exposed to far more toxins than ever before, our food quality is diminishing, we eat on the run preventing us from chewing food properly, stress levels are at an all-time high which impacts our ability to secrete digestive acids. As a result, we're not digesting our food properly, becoming more nutritionally depleted, and are completely disconnected from our gut!

Have you ever experienced bloating or cramping but you couldn't work out what was causing it or what actually relieved it, because it seemed like every day it was different, one day you could eat bread no worries, the next it sat in your gut like a brick? Then some days your poos are frequent and loose, but then you can't seem to go for days! This is the modern-day 'gut' pandemic; not knowing exactly what eases your discomfort and feeling like you're chasing your tail when it comes to uncovering the causes of the gas! Understanding the digestive system can be a complex task with the many elements all with their own unique roles in the digestion process, resulting in confusion and sometimes hopelessness.

One of the most common complaints women with hormonal imbalances and conditions of the reproductive system complain of is extreme bloating to the point they feel and look six months pregnant. Now let me take you back to where it all began and highlight the importance of being in tune with your body and connected enough to feel what's happening at a cellular level, because what can start as a tiny 'hole' will quickly spread to an unmanageable gape if nothing is done to address the cause of the friction. What can start off as a minor irritation will soon spread like wildfire if it is not repaired quickly.

Kelly, aged 22 presented with extreme abdominal cramping that was so severe she ended up in emergency, only to be told it was trapped wind (farts). Awkward. However, the pain was so crippling and frequent that it was really affecting her work productivity and ability to enjoy life. The problem was there was no pattern as to what would trigger an 'attack', so every day felt like a game of Russian Roulette, robbing her of her desire to enjoy food or eating out.

Kelly had a typical 'standard Australian diet'. She believed she ate well. She always chose wholemeal or seeded bread over white, ate salads where she could, stuck to one cup of coffee a day with lactose-free milk, no sugar and kept her sweets to a moderate intake. She ate lean meat twice a day and restricted her pasta intake even though she loved carbs, because she was aware too many 'made her fat'.

Leaky gut syndrome

One of the major causes of a dysfunctional digestive system is inflammation as a result of repeatedly eating irritative foods which contain proteins that the human body does not often tolerate well. The top five culprits are alcohol, coffee, refined sugar, gluten, and dairy as well as compounds such as pharmaceutical medications which will degrade the quality of the digestive tissue over time.

'Leaky gut' occurs when the cells lining your stomach become damaged due to the constant irritation and exposure to these items. Remember I told you about the body's innate ability to heal itself? When any human tissue is damaged, the body quickly responds by increasing the blood flow to the site delivering inflammatory mediators to initiate the repair process, immune cells to clear up the damaged cells and extra nutrients to rapidly repair the damage. But it's like anything in life, if we keep abusing it, eventually it will wear out and become irreparable. This is what happens when the body is smashed with irritative foods on a daily basis over a long period of time. You won't feel any symptoms for a long time as your body's clean-up process is so effective, but eventually the body will start to feel the burden, and so will you.

This chronic inflammatory-immune response occurring through the gut healing process then leads to the development of allergies and food intolerances, by which partially digested proteins now slip through the gaps in the stomach lining into the bloodstream where they shouldn't be, alerting the immune system, which quickly identifies the undigested foods as foreign bodies, eliciting an immune response to attack. Our very clever immune system then recognises this antigen immune complex, creating the same inflammatory immune response every time you are in contact with the allergen. So, depending on the individual, this may present as sneezing, a runny nose, watery eyes, headache, low mood, low energy, skin rash or any of the many ways that food intolerances physically manifest in the body.

This prolonged exposure to inflammatory substances most likely started at around age 4-6 months upon the ingestion of your first solid food. The general paediatric recommendations from the medical industry are to start infants on grains, which I strongly disagree with. Introducing foods to an underdeveloped digestive system will always place too much burden on the body, but that's a story for another time. Formula-fed babies are also exposed to this same inflammatory response due to the cow's milk and additives in processed formulas.

After many years we eventually end up with a mildly ulcerated and inflamed digestive tract, which is now unable to repair itself on its own. Upon ingestion of anything evenly slightly complex to digest you may or may not experience aching in the abdominal area, and with the hyper-stimulated immune activity occurring, nasty bacteria is now left largely unchecked and able to multiply more easily than normal. We're exposed to bad bacteria everywhere, which is usually not a big deal with a fully functioning immune system quickly eradicating it before it can breed. On top of this we now have compromised circulation to the digestive system due to the chronic inflammation and a stressed digestive system in general, which when lacking healthy blood flow, adequate nutrient delivery and vitality is now losing its ability to produce adequate amounts of hydrochloric acid, teamed with the immune system that isn't functioning optimally, allowing those bad bacteria to duplicate and build in number.

Due to the enormity of people suffering in this nature through their digestive systems, food intolerance testing has become popular, however, I'm a believer that is can be an unnecessary, costly exercise and encourages a very fragmented approach to healing your tummy problems. Eliminating natural wholefoods because the digestive system doesn't have the capacity to effectively break down and process them properly is missing the mark by a long shot. If you are reacting to natural whole foods, then the work needs to be done on repairing the leaky gut, restoring digestive secretions and modulating that hyper-stimulated 'allergic' immune reaction.

This is the difference once again between treating at a symptomatic surface level and addressing the issues holistically by treating the cause of the problems. Like any situation, there will always be a time and a place to have this $300-400 test performed, but if you are not healing the system and merely cutting out foods, you will never change your situation. There are more effective ways to support the digestive system including elimination diets and the blood type diet to get you started on healing your system, which I believe is more financially viable and a more holistic approach which empowers the sufferer to actually take charge of their own healing journey.

Back to Kelly. Her symptoms continued to worsen. Now not only was she experiencing severe cramping, she often had a sore, dull ache in the abdomen area and loads of foul-smelling gas to contend with. The growth of the bad bacteria was increasing, creating dysbiosis (an imbalanced gut microbiome ruled by bad bacteria in the absence of healthy bacteria) which produce gases of their own, causing the bloating and off-smelling wind. Dysbiosis, also known as small intestinal bacterial overgrowth (SIBO) and treating this phenomenon is a pivotal part of overall health and wellness and prevention of chronic disease, especially auto-immune conditions and endometriosis, cysts and fibroids.

And with the increased pressure through the digestive system, this muscle was losing tone and strength by the day as well as the ability to produce optional amounts of digestive acids to break down her food, which meant her meals just seemed to sit in her gut and ferment. Motility then becomes an issue, with the digestive muscles losing tone, resulting in further bloating, constipation, inflammation, and the cycle continues.

Now with the inflammation, dysbiosis and under-production of digestive acids, the environment was far less than perfect for maintaining a healthy gut microbiome and all strains of beneficial bacteria began to slowly decline. A healthy gut houses billions of beneficial bacteria which work to boost your immune system, organise your hormones, assist with communication from the brain to the rest of the body, and assist with maintaining a healthy, happy mood. Without the presence of these happy helpers, this meant further issues for Kelly's digestion - more pain, bloating, gas and now changes to her bowel movements, fluctuating from diarrhoea to constipation, depending what she ate or how badly inflamed the gut was on that particular day.

With food sitting in her stomach for hours upon hours, she felt uncomfortable from the moment she ate in the mornings and soon developed bouts of acid reflux as her food fermented and easily regurgitated up the oesophagus. Kelly's energy levels declined; she became more nutritionally depleted due to not being able to extract nutrients from the foods she was eating. Months and months passed with no improvement, despite cutting out as many foods as she possibly could and self-prescribing herself an over the counter probiotic.

Kelly now avoided social events involving food and she was unable to feel comfortable in her clothing as her permanently bloated waistline looked more and more like she was expecting. A completely dysfunctional digestive system and next to no beneficial bacteria also meant Kelly was no longer metabolising and eliminating her hormones correctly each month and so her system began to accumulate exogenous environmental oestrogens, messing with her cycle. Premenstrually she felt even more bloated, depressed, snappy and her bleed was becoming more painful and heavier than ever. On top of this, she seemed to get sick or have a cold sore outbreak before each period, with her immune system continuing to struggle.

Kelly visited her GP who referred her for scans and a colonoscopy, which revealed nothing, and she was sent away with a diagnosis of irritable bowel syndrome, a prescription for anti-depressants and an antacid tablet.

The problem with medical screening regarding the digestive system is that, unless they can see a tangible 'disease', like a growth or severe ulceration of the colon, they can't actually measure the functionality of the digestive system which means everything can look normal, despite being far from healthy. When Kelly finally came to see me in the clinic, she was exhausted, depressed and lacking any motivation or hope for improvement.

The Gluten Debate

Gluten and gluten intolerance is very much a hot topic nowadays and with the awareness surrounding the negative implications on the digestive system growing, it's inevitable to stir controversy and discussion among the medical industry and make for some prime media coverage! Gluten, or more specifically gliadin, which is the inflammatory protein found in popular grains such as wheat, rye, barley and spelt is hard to resist for many, after all it is this component which gives bread that delicious soft fluffy texture.

Gluten wasn't always the baddie, however, over the years with increasing agricultural development, the involvement of genetic modifications, overuse of industrial herbicides and pesticides, gluten has become something everyone needs to be wary of, due to the natural adaptation process which has rendered this protein undigestible and inflammatory to the human gut. Many people are now under the impression that unless you have been diagnosed with Celiac disease, an inflammatory auto-immune condition by which gluten triggers an immune response that damages the lining of the small intestine you do not need to worry about gluten.

However, the reality is, gluten is inflammatory. Think of it like glass. If you swallowed glass it's going to cut and damage your intestinal lining, regardless as to whether you're allergic to it or not. Now this may seem like a dramatic comparison, but there is much evidence to prove that over time the inflammatory nature of gluten will damage and destroy your intestinal lining which leads to the interference of nutrient absorption, causing a whole host of symptoms. The only difference is, someone who doesn't have an allergy isn't going to notice the damage immediately as would some with clinically diagnosed Celiac disease. But it's this long term slow and steady degradation of the gut and subsequent microbiome which has the dramatic effect on your health leading to inflammatory conditions such as joint pain, nerve damage, migraines, thyroid destruction, infertility and the downward spiral continues.

Gluten sensitivity, which I believe everyone will develop eventually from ingesting the inflammatory protein, has been associated with depression and anxiety due to the damage in the brain-gut connection and resultant diminishing of the microbiome, causing problems which affects neurotransmitter production and signalling, affecting mood and energy levels and creating systemic inflammation exacerbating arthritic pain, and eventually triggering underlying auto-immune conditions including Hashimoto's thyroiditis. This occurs because the gliadin protein molecule of gluten closely resembles thyroid antibodies, which elicits in auto-immune response on the gland. When gliadin breaches the protective barrier of the gut and enters the bloodstream, the immune system tags it for destruction. The same anti-gliadin antibodies produced in response to the gliadin once it's entered our bloodstream directly mimic antibodies produced by the thyroid, which can lead to an increased immune attack on the thyroid gland.

Signs you might be intolerant to gluten will eventually show up as:

- Fluid retention
- Skin rashes
- Fatigue
- Aching joints
- Brain fog
- Irritability
- Puffy eyes or dark circles under your eyes
- Frequent colds and flu
- Anxiety
- Headaches
- Hay fever symptoms

The damaging effects of gluten are widespread because once the damage to the gut is done, the undigested gliadin protein is able to escape into the blood stress and cause havoc wherever it travels.

Repairing the digestive system

When it comes to repairing the digestive system, there's a step-by-step process that must be followed, and all elements of this fine-tuned machine must be addressed, or the cycle of poor health and digestion will continue. This is where most motivated health enthusiasts go wrong, throwing themselves into Google and the easily-accessible array of health supplements at your local pharmacy, set about on a mission to fix their health problems. But if we don't address all of the elements Kelly and many more of you are experiencing, that tiny little niggle will continue to grow into a monster.

Step 1 - Cleanse the colon
As addressed in Chapter 6, this is a crucial step which can't be avoided. It's about clearing out that inhospitable environment that the bad bugs are utilising to multiply and making way for a microbiome that thrives!

Step 2 – Eradicate dysbiotic flora (bad bugs, parasites and foreign invaders)
This has been discussed previously in Chapter 7. Skipping this step will prevent restoring digestive health and ultimately overall wellbeing.

Step 3 – Remove the top five inflammatory foods
If you keep scratching off the 'scab,' how will the wound heal? This is how your stomach feels when you keep exposing it to the top five inflammatory culprits: coffee, alcohol, refined sugar, dairy, gluten. I highly recommend you set yourself up on an elimination diet with your trusty journal or attempt the blood group diet based on your blood type. This is very much a broad approach to 'eating right' for your body and as much as I see the benefits of the blood type diet, it is still very much a one-size-fits-all approach and certainly doesn't apply to everyone. It is, however, a great starting place for reducing irritative foods from your diet while you are starting the repair process and learning how to listen to your body. More of that in Chapter 10.

Action
Get yourself a diet diary or journal to start recording your meals and subsequent reactions and feelings following each meal.

Cut out the top five inflammatory foods. If this is overwhelming, start slowly with one food at a time.

Step 4 – Stimulate digestive secretions
Digestive enzymes, bile and hydrochloric acid can all be classified as digestive secretions and are required for digesting food, breaking up waste, supporting the immune function and also clearing excess mucus and foreign matter from your system. When we are not digesting our food properly due to an underproduction of digestive secretions common symptoms due to eating the wrong foods, stress, other elements of the digestive system being clogged up, like your gallbladder or bowel, the liver being sluggish, medication reactions and so forth your body will start to experience bloating, reflux, indigestion, abdominal distension, pain, burping, gas and general uncomfortable feelings.

Digestive bitters and essential oils
This is my preferred method of action because bitters such as gentian root, angelica, bitter orange, slippery elm, artichoke leaf, cardamom seed, milk thistle, cinnamon, ginger root, galangal root, dandelion and burdock stimulate the body's natural production of digestive secretions and is thus a holistic approach to restoring function, rather than relying on an external substance to take over the digestive process, as you'll see with acids. This also includes essential oils such as anise seed, peppermint, ginger, caraway seed, coriander seed, tarragon, and fennel seed, which will work quickly to soothe an upset tummy, although I do not recommend consuming essential oils internally as an ongoing process. This practice is safer when applied topically over the abdomen or painful area using a carrier oil.

Celery juice
I'm sharing this from the book 'Medical Medium', by Anthony William. He's an incredible healer. If you ever get a chance to check out his books, I highly recommend them.

Celery juice contains unique sodium molecules and mineral salts and nutrients, which have the ability to restore your stomach's hydrochloric acid production. The only thing I will say about this protocol is that it will have a cooling effect on the system, which is great if your liver is hot and angry like most of you, but if you naturally have a weak, cold constitution, celery juice may create other problems in your system, so like everything, it's about how it makes your individual body feel, not what is working for everyone else.

Juice fresh celery daily – approximately 200-250ml (1 cup) and drink every morning, first thing in the morning on an empty stomach. Do not add other fruits or vegetables, it is very important to have the celery completely on its own. You can include the celery leaves if desired, these have a lovely diuretic effect on the body and can be great for flushing out fluid retention and is very supportive of your kidney health, however these do have a bitter taste.

Apple cider vinegar
As a general rule, apple cider vinegar (ACV) is quite acidic and abrasive to the gut and not something I recommend using ongoing for an extended period of time, but in the short term while your body is still requiring help with its digestion, shotting some diluted ACV can help create the necessary acid balance in your gut to assist with breaking down your food.

Dilute 15-20ml of ACV with a little water and take this either just before eating, while you are eating or straight after eating. Quite often acid reflux is caused by an under-production of acid in your stomach, so experiment with taking the ACV at different times. If you take it before eating and find your reflux gets worse, then the cause of your acid reflux is most likely due to an over-production of acid. If it soothes the problem, then your reflux and indigestion are most likely caused by an underproduction of acid.

Lemon juice
Squeeze fresh lemon juice into a glass of lukewarm water and drink first thing every morning to stimulate the liver and digestive secretions.

Keep in mind lemon juice is very acidic, which is why it assists with your digestion, so if it starts to irritate your teeth and deplete the enamel, drink your lemon water through a straw.

Another thing worth noticing is that the only reason lemon has a counter-alkalising effect on the body is because the acidity stimulates the pancreas to release a whole heap of enzymes and buffering ions to counteract the acidity, resulting in an alkaline environment. Long term use of lemon juice in the absence of a healthy supportive diet including foods and herbs which support the pancreas can deplete your pancreatic enzymes, so this is not a method I recommend ongoing and daily for the rest of your life.

Consume foods with naturally occurring digestive enzymes
Pineapple, papaya/paw paw, bee pollen or fermented foods such as sauerkraut, kim chi, kombucha.

Step 5 – Soothe the stomach
This is the healing process of the gut which aims to soothe the inflammation and damage done to the digestive tract through the ingestion of inflammatory substances. This includes the use of natural herbal supplements and foods which have a healing effect on the lining of the gut and intestinal tract and will best support the healing process if carried out consistently over an extended period of time while avoiding the irritants.

Slippery elm
My favourite anti-inflammatory gut-healing herb which soothes and supports the natural mucus membrane. This is great made into a tea, sweetened with manuka honey which has its own demulcent healing properties on the gut and drunk on an empty stomach morning and night. To improve the taste, try adding ginger and licorice powder, which also heal the gut.

Gut healing tonic
This is a lovely start to the day. Add turmeric powder, cinnamon and manuka honey to boiling water and drink as a morning elixir, or added to your favourite herbal tea, rooibos and ginger are great.

Vegetable broth
You've more than likely heard of the gut-healing benefits of bone broth due to its high content of collagen, but I personally am not a fan of using animal products which are acidic and increase urea in our bodies. Vegetable broth, on the other hand, has the same anti-inflammatory healing properties and natural collagen content to support gut healing. This can be consumed like a morning cup of soup on an empty stomach. Collect all your vegetable scraps in a container and store them in the freezer until you have collected a large amount. Then simply add these to a pot of boiling water or a slow cooker and combine with fresh herbs such as parsley, garlic, bay leaves, basil, thyme and rosemary to increase the therapeutic properties and improve the flavour.

Step 6 – Include prebiotics for healthy GIT microflora in your diet

Prebiotics are derived from specific fibres and provide an important food or fuel source for our microbiome. This helps the gut bacteria produce nutrients for your colon cells and leads to a healthier digestive system. Some of these nutrients include short-chain fatty acids like butyrate, acetate and propionate. Probiotics WILL NOT colonise, unless they are given at the same time as prebiotics, which is another reason why people waste their money self-prescribing probiotics.

The top prebiotic containing foods:
- Chicory root
- Dandelion greens
- Jerusalem artichoke
- Garlic
- Onion
- Leek
- Asparagus
- Bananas
- Barley
- Oats
- Apples
- Konjac root
- Cacao

- Burdock root
- Flaxseeds
- Seaweed
- Yacon root
- Wheat bran

Step 7 – Stimulate the gall bladder

Your gall bladder stores bile which is required to help us emulsify fats in our diet. It drains waste products from the liver into the small intestine so they can be eliminated and assists with the absorption of fat-soluble vitamins - A, D, E and K - as well as many other lipid-soluble nutrients and antioxidants.

When food enters the small intestine, a hormone called cholecystokinin is released which signals the gall bladder to contract and release bile into the small intestine through the common bile duct. If your diet is high in fat processed fats, animal fats and trans fatty acids, which are difficult to digest, they start to build up in your system, creating a sticky mess, which eventually hardens. Bilirubin is a by-product of red blood cell recycling and it can also build up if our liver function is sluggish and then we have bile salts, which if they build up all of these things harden and lead to gallstones forming.

Gallstones are generally small, hard deposits inside the gall bladder that are formed when stored bile crystallises. Anyone who has ever enjoyed some greasy fish and chips a few times in their lifetime will no doubt have accumulated cholesterol stones. I'd say nearly everyone has lots of these little cholesterol or gallstones, but it's not until they become a certain size that you will experience pain. Coffee enemas or gall bladder flushes using herbs, citrus fruits and apples are the best way to clear them out, before they increase in size and cause damage!

A gall bladder attack can be very debilitating, however, the medical approach to cut out this organ is both dangerous in the long term and naïve to think our body will thrive without it. Restoring the function and repairing the damage will always be a better approach than removing something that cannot be put back. This is a huge part of changing the culture and belief that our 'body is misbehaving' when we experience pain and discomfort. Your body is actually just communicating with you and letting it know that something is wrong, and it needs help. Simply ignoring the issues by 'cutting' out a natural organ will only lead to the stress being diverted to another area of the body and like the domino effect, what is set in motion can have a devastating widespread effect on the overall functioning of the human body.

The GIT microbiome
It has been said that humans contain more beneficial live bacteria within our entire system than we do DNA, so as imagined, this bacteria plays huge roles in the assistance of a healthy human body. This includes:

- Aiding digestion
- Detoxification and elimination of toxins - especially the metabolism of oestrogen
- Supporting the immune system
- Stabilising mental and emotional wellbeing
- Signalling to various cells and neurotransmitters.

However, if your diet is high in processed sugar or alcohol, you're stressed or taking medications such as antibiotics or the oral contraceptive pill, or you have an underlying infection, dysbiosis or parasite, your microbiome will diminish.

Step 8 – Replenish GIT Microflora with Probiotics
Probiotics are live beneficial bacteria or yeasts which support your health, especially your gut health and digestion. There are millions of different strains with plenty still yet to be identified and researched, but these friendly invaders live symbiotically within our gastrointestinal tract improving our health, emotional wellbeing and hormone balance. For this reason, taking a probiotic supplement can be highly advantageous but doing so without first cleaning up the environment and eradicating it of harmful foreign invaders is like pouring water into a leaky bucket. A big waste of time.

Probiotics occur naturally in our foods, with the best sources being from freshly grown fruits and vegetables which should be eaten before washing these valuable bacteria off their surface. Another great reason to buy pesticide-free produce from your local farmer's market.

Fermented foods are another source; however, this is far from a one-size-fits-all winning formula. Fermented foods are high in histamines which can cause more harm than good in a sensitive system by which the natural flora is out of balance and there's dysbiotic flora. So, before experimenting with things like kombucha, kim chi, kefir and sauerkraut, make sure you implement steps 1 to 8 of this protocol or you will just add to the 'shit storm' that's already occurring in your guts and have yourself feeling worse for it.

Step 9 – Retrain the bowel

See Chapter 6 for the bowel retrain protocol. Ensure you get your bowels to a standard of a minimum of two movements per day to ensure healthy toxin elimination, hormone regulation and maintaining a home for the microbiome to thrive in. Check out https://balancedbabes.net/bowelretrain/

Step 5 - Supporting Gut & Digestive Health

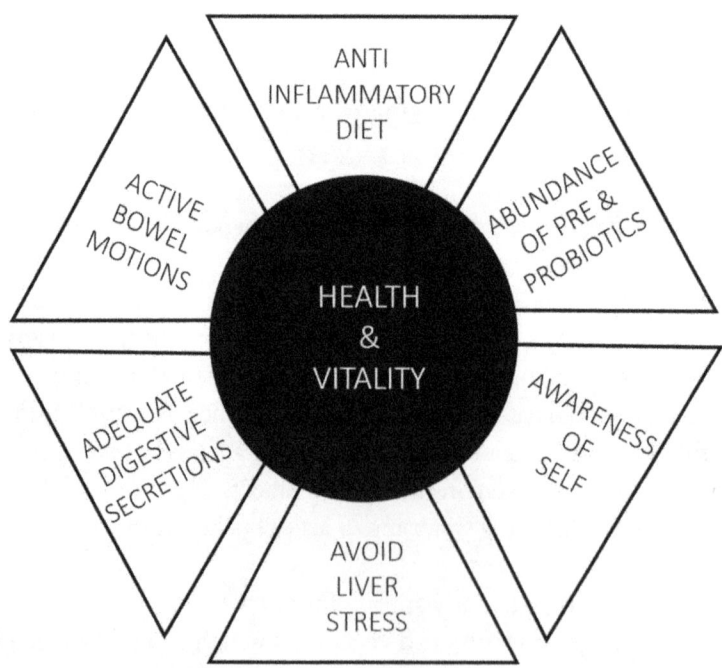

A Gut Feeling

We've all experienced it before, that gut feeling that something is just not quite right, even though you can't consciously put your finger on it. It's an uncomfortable feeling and inner knowing that something needs addressing. Be it your intuition or an irking gut feeling, your gut really is your guru when it comes to all-knowing and understanding of the human body, your health and what your body requires. If we can learn to tap into this feeling and listen, we develop a deep connection with our cells and can start to understand what our body requires to thrive. Although this may seem farfetched without a degree in anatomy and some extensive investigation tests, there truly is nothing that your doctor or naturopath can tell you about your health that your body doesn't already know and isn't already trying to communicate with you through symptom.

Spiritual shape-up

Connecting with your gut and strengthening your intuition

A big part of this comes down to accepting that everything you experience is happening for a reason, as a consequence or reaction to the way we are living our life or even our subconscious beliefs. There is no such thing as coincidence, only reactions for every action, so tuning in to your body, practising self-inquiry and consciously connecting the dots as to how our everyday actions are affecting our health is a huge part of living life which is supportive of your personal health.

What is your gut trying to tell you?
- Learn to quieten the analytical mind – go within, practices stillness and meditation
- Ask questions – self-enquiry
- Journal your answers
- Take aligned action based on your thoughts
- Back yourself – trust your intuition.

Journaling the journey

Make a list of 3-5 things which excite you. This could be people you love, places or food. Then make a list of 3-5 things that you don't trust, enjoy or are afraid of.

Close your eyes and picture these things. Spend a few minutes in the vibration and fantasy of the things that excite you and notice how that makes your body and your energy feel. Now focus on the negative things you thought of. Feel how your body contracts and a prickly feeling rolls over your body. Practice identifying these sensations and connecting with your 'gut feelings' in everyday situations.

When you experience situations that have a negative effect on you, make a point of journaling about this once you hop into bed that night. Recognise the subtle information and feelings we have access to when we are still enough, self-aware enough and paying attention to our energy and vibration.

CHAPTER 10

NAILING NUTRITION

"The food you eat can be either the safest and most powerful form of medicine or the slowest form of poison."

Sara Gottfried

This chapter is about nailing nutrition, understanding what you specifically need to thrive and learning how to listen to your body's cues so you can choose a style of eating which truly supports your health and wellbeing. Because what is right for that cover girl model or even what a dietitian has suggested rarely actually meets your individual body's needs.

As profound as science can be, when it comes to measuring human health, it is extremely limited and always skewed by individual perception and understanding. Health cannot be measured by how we look, how well we perform on an academic test or an athletic tract, and to simply base it upon how we function and feel is still at best limited when we look at the complexity of the emotional, spiritual, mental and physical diversities of the human body. The power of our innate knowing or 'gut feeling' will always override what science can measure within a randomised clinical trial, especially when the individual is connected to their body and has a true understanding of what good health feels like.

So, what exactly is nutrition? The most common mistake people make when fuelling their bodies is not understanding what the body actually requires to function. Nutrition and diet are two completely different things, but unfortunately are perceived as the same, which is why many people fail to thrive when selecting eating plans based on an external recommendation. Think of it this way, if you want your car to run well or even work for you, it's simple. Make sure it's got fuel in it and get it serviced regularly and your car will do what it is meant to do for you; get you from A to B. In a way your body is kinda the same; if you don't fuel it correctly, it will break down and understanding what fuel, aka 'nutrition' is going to give your 'body' the best performance is like knowing whether to fuel your car with petrol or diesel, both equally effective fuel types in different engines.

Nutrition, according to the English Oxford dictionary is the process of providing or obtaining the food necessary for health and growth. And if we break that down further, it's the fuel each and every living cell in our body requires to carry out the thousands of functions which need to occur within our tissues every day to keep us alive.

Nutrition can be broken into macronutrients and micronutrients. For macronutrients, think 'large'. This is very much the broad fuel types; carbohydrates, fats and proteins which our bodies need to function. These are the 'key' energy sources which fuel our body. Micronutrients are smaller, more intricate nutrients including the minerals, vitamins and phytonutrients which all play specific roles in catalysing specific biological functions within our cells. A diet focused purely on macronutrients with little consideration of that food's micronutrient content is like having a lock with the wrong key; you're not going to get to where you want without both elements.

In the dieting world, unfortunately a large focus is on macronutrients and their measurements of energy, particularly in regards to calories burnt versus calories consumed. This typically ignores the food source's micronutrient content, which will always have dangerous health implications that will catch up with you eventually.

Micronutrient importance is completely undervalued when it comes to health based on a one-size-fits-all 'dietary' model focusing on what the average male or female needs according to their weight and age alone. Micronutrients are the catalyst to every biological change that occurs in the human body, which of course differs greatly from one person to the next, based on changing environmental factors and lifestyle practices. Focusing on 'macros' without giving a thought to 'micros' is very much the difference between 'existing' versus 'thriving'. Ensuring you have as many micronutrients in your body as possible, every single day, is the key to living with vitality and longevity. It is as simple as, what you put in your body matters and has a direct effect on your health.

Sadly, in 2014 I attended a prominent cancer hospital in Victoria due to my father's diagnosis of stage 4 Melanoma. It was a heartbreaking reality check to see posters plastered all around the hospital, celebrating the fact that they now offered Tim Tams, Twisties and 2-minute noodles to their patients, as if it were a good thing. It was at that moment I realised the overwhelming disconnect between understanding the power of food as medicine and human health within our medical industry and the kamikaze mission these cancer patients were facing while their immune systems were being suppressed with chemotherapy drugs and the cancer cells fuelled like petrol on fire with processed sugary foods.

And although the awareness is growing steadily, with amazing advocates of whole food nutrition sharing their wisdom such as Don and Tyler Tolman, David Wolfe, and Anthony William, the power of nutrition and plant-based medicine is increasing, but it still blows my mind how little attention is given to food and its impact on our bodies by the medical system. And for how far advanced we are with science and medical intervention, the basic fundamentals of nutrition are still ignored when it comes to healing the human body.

There are literally hundreds of different eating styles, plans and diets out there, some which are 'scientifically proven' with the latest research suggesting this is what the human body must consume, but the truth is, there is no one diet that fits all and certainly not when you think about the diversity in the human body from one person to the next. We cannot deny the wisdom of mother nature and the gifts she has supplied for human consumption, providing key nutritional value for health, and at some point, common sense must contend with science to bring about our own innate knowing. Humans naively believing they know better than mother nature is the ultimate demise when it comes to human health.

Factors which are going to influence what is the 'right' eating plan for you include:

- Your current state of health
- Genetic predispositions
- The amount of stress in your life
- The stage of your reproductive years: menstruating, pregnancy, lactating, menopausal
- The health of your immune system
- Your predisposition to allergies
- Your gut health
- Your liver health
- Blood group
- Current nutritional deficiencies
- Health of your adrenal system
- Body type
- Level of activity
- Lifestyle
- Age
- Gender
- Level of muscle mass
- Spiritual beliefs
- Tastebuds
- Personality

Assuming that there is one type of diet out there that everyone should follow for good health is at best naïve and extremely dangerous. The only way to understand what truly works best for you specifically is trial and error, which is fast-tracked when we get back into our body and start to listen and feel how our body is responding.

My 'dietary' journey

There was a period in my life, for quite a few years to be honest, where I consumed a block of Cadbury chocolate a day. Except not many knew because I did it in hiding. It came with so much shame and self-judgement, especially since I was a 'degree-qualified nutritionist' who should have known better.

Living with a food addiction may seem trivial, it's hardly 'life-threatening', I mean I could financially support my habit and I wasn't hurting anyone in the process, so I suffered in silence for many years, secretly loathing myself and physically cringing every time I looked at my body in a mirror. What I was experiencing seemed minor in comparison to families dealing with drug and alcohol abuse, which is exactly why it is a problem which affects so many people, gradually declining their health and self-esteem over the years.

From a 'diagnostic' point of view, I never truly struggled with my weight, it was more my warped perception of my body. The heaviest I ever weighed was 13kg heavier than my current weight, which certainly didn't classify me as morbidly obese. I hated the way I looked and as a result I was constantly searching for that magic pill or diet that would change me forever. I didn't just hate how I looked, I hated who I was, I hated that food consumed my every waking thought and I hated how out of control I felt. As much as I loved the taste of chocolate and the quick hit I received each time I indulged, chocolate was actually a form of punishment, because I was never satisfied by the sweet taste, so I always ate until I felt sick and felt even more disgusted about my body. Food became an obsession, constantly restricting myself, making new rules about what I could and couldn't consume, trying every new fad diet as it presented on social media but never actually feeling like my body shape was changing, because my perception of myself never actually changed.

The one thing about this journey was that it meant I spent years trying every different eating plan under the sun and over time I learnt to understand what actually made me feel good physically. It's been years in the making mastering where I am now and actually learning to love my figure, and the only way I was able to master my relationship with food was to master my relationship with myself. Once I was able to love and accept myself for me and truly understand who I was, what I stood for and what actually felt good in my body, I was able to feel more, which allowed me to recognise the impact different foods had on my mood, my weight and my health. My journey to 'nailing nutrition' was very much physical body awareness and deep emotional healing. That part you'll master in the next chapter!

The biggest take-away I can share from my journey was how I went wrong when choosing my fuel source, because I was only ever focused on what effect it was going to have on my body shape. I only cared if the food was going to help me lose weight, not if it was going to help my health, something I was forced to look at when my health hit an all-time low. The body has an amazing way of showing you what you refuse to see if you continue to ignore it, which is exactly what happened when I was diagnosed as starting menopause at age 27.

I was so disconnected from how the food actually made me feel or whether or not it actually benefited my health, that I was oblivious to the fact I never really had optimal energy levels, I suffered from eczema on and off since childhood and despite always choosing to adopt a positive 'glass half full' attitude to life, I was suffering from depression more than not. And my diet definitely played a huge role in all of this.

NAILING NUTRITION

The process of learning what diet is right for you

It all starts with being present and practising mindfulness when you're eating. Eating on the run or completely distracted from the actual process and reason as to WHY you are actually eating is one of the major issues which disconnects us from the effect food has on our body. One of the easiest ways to start making connections with what your body is relaying after meals is to start keeping a diet diary. Expect to be keeping a record like this for at least 6-12 weeks, which might sound like a massive pain in the butt, but the power of the information you will obtain by learning what your body actually likes and what is the ultimate best fuel for you is priceless.

You are unique. There is not one other person who is built anything like you or has anything even close to your specific genetic makeup. Your body has its own unique requirements which are different to everyone else, so trying a diet purely because it worked for someone else isn't enough of an indicator it's the answer for you. There are many great teachers who share varying philosophies about what foods heal or harm the body. There's so much variation in the information shared regarding meal sizes, the best times to eat, fasting, carb loading, high protein, low fat, high fat, organic, vegan, plant-based, low fruit and so forth, and with the information being largely contradicting, you will need to learn how to adopt the gems from all of these 'dietary' guidelines, from every book you read, every podcast you hear or class you take and individually apply them to your lifestyle and your physical body. This requires patience, testing, feeling and then making an in-tune, educated decision about what feels right for your body. This may take years to master but is nonetheless an obligation you have, to listen and find out what your body needs for you to feel and look your best.

Your diet and food choices have a powerful effect on all elements of your life. Not just your physical appearance or your physical health. It also shapes who you are as a person and helps us to align with our soul tribe. When I started following a plant-based diet, I connected with the most amazing friends who have opened up my world to many new adventures and helped me to develop an even deeper understanding of who I am, finding my truth. Food is powerful, as medicine and as a means of connecting and sharing with others.

Key signs from your body your diet isn't right for you

- Inflammation – fluid retention, aching joints, bones and muscles
- Deficiencies – changes to your hair skin and nails including weird markings, rashes, damage to nails, changes to appearance and structure of nails, coatings on the tongue, weak hair and nails
- Frequent infections – feeling run down and constantly fighting off infections, picking up everything that's going around the office or daycare centre
- Mood swings
- Poor performance - low energy, poor recovery post-exercise or 'binge drinking sessions' (bad hangovers)
- Weight that will not budge.

Healing crisis

Also known as a Herxheimer reaction, a healing crisis is a natural process triggered by the release of endotoxins. These reactions occur more commonly and more severely in those suffering from chronic illness and as the body begins to restore health and balance by removing toxins or bacteria which have been blocking the body's ability to heal itself. When we make healthy changes to our diet and start to consume less processed foods which have been burdening the liver and organs and eat more nutrient-rich fruits and vegetables, the body will naturally start to release stored toxins or bacteria which in itself can result in uncomfortable sensations such as:

- Headaches
- Aching joints
- Bloating

- Changes to bowels
- Low energy and low mood

This can quite often be confused as believing you are having an allergic reaction or intolerance to a healthy food. It is actually the complete opposite, which is why you should take your time when experimenting with new foods and not write anything off until you have trailed it for 6-12 weeks. This rule only applies to fruits and vegetables, anything processed or of animal origin will never have a 'healing crisis' effect on the body, so if you experience these symptoms after consuming animal products such as meat, eggs or dairy that is an immediate reaction from that food group.

Fruits and vegetables are mother nature's gift and have the ability to heal the body. Some people truly believe that if you are having an allergic reaction to a fruit or vegetable which leads to extreme discomfort, it is just an extreme release of endotoxins which will eventually stop as you consistently consume the food causing the reaction. This of course is a theory that needs to be approached with caution, especially if you have an anaphylactic reaction, but I do truly believe that the fault lies within your immune system and digestive system as well as the underlying infection and toxicity build-up in the organ which is reacting and not the result of a fruit or vegetable causing harm in your body.

To meat or not to meat

Meat consumption is undoubtedly the most controversial food group in terms of supporting arguments for and against the health benefits of consuming animal flesh. Meat should be the first thing you set about experimenting with if you are currently a meat eater and open to testing if this is truly healing or harming your body. As a non-meat eater, I have chosen to avoid eating animals because of the complexity in breaking down this tissue and the debatable question as to whether or not we actually absorb and assimilate the protein and minerals found in animal flesh.

When I was following the popular paleo diet and eating two serves of meat a day, I weighed 8-10kg more than my current weight. I looked bloated and inflamed and my face was a lot rounder than it is now. In theory, the paleo diet is a fantastic way of eating; it educates people to avoid processed packaged foods, mucus-forming dairy products and is anti-inflammatory due to the avoidance of grains. All of this is backed by scientific evidence which suggests it is a suitable way of eating based on the diet our ancestors consumed in the primal era. This style of eating has gained huge traction with many benefits among those who suffer from inflammatory auto-immune conditions dramatically reducing joint pain, inflammation and chronic disease, but it's not necessarily for everyone.

As a child I never enjoyed eating meat, in fact I hated it, but was able to force myself to eat chicken and the occasional 'spag bol' disguising the meat with as much Napoli sauce and vegetables as possible so I couldn't actually taste or sense the texture of the meat. I chose to experiment with a paleo lifestyle because I wanted to lose weight. At the time I was suffering from adrenal fatigue and had put on weight quickly, so my ability to listen and feel what my body was telling me was severely clouded by my desire to lose weight. Within a short amount of time my digestive issues began. I quite often felt bloated and gassy. I craved sugars, especially chocolate because I was depriving myself of complex carbohydrates and my whole body was riddled with eczema.

Due to my blood group, type A, and my inability to produce high amounts of stomach acid, my body was unable to process the meat effectively, which meant I wasn't actually breaking down and absorbing the minerals from the animal proteins, my liver was becoming more and more burdened and I was carrying an extra 8kg of body fat as a result. Truth be told, I was far from a picture of health, but I continued on this eating style for a good 18 months because all the books I was reading said this was the way we should be eating. I wasn't listening to my body, despite the signals it was giving me. It doesn't matter how scientifically sound or how well the dietitian or nutritionist can rationalise It, if it's not the right eating plan for you, you are not going to feel your best. And your body is going to let you know, through physical feelings, aka symptoms!

Meat is one of those things that works for some but not for many, and for those who do thrive on animal proteins, I still believe over-consumption is a big issue, including portion sizes and the number of serves consumed per week. Meat is still very congesting on the digestive system and creates a lot of acidity in the body, so it should always be consumed in moderation if you do choose to eat meat. Start by experimenting with reduced portion sizes of just 100g per meal. Limit your intake to just once per day and experiment with vegetarian days. Use your diet diary to determine how you are feeling following your changes and always persevere beyond the first four weeks as detoxification symptoms are likely to occur once you reduce your intake of animal proteins and the liver is able to remove more toxins.

Check in with yourself at the end of each day.

- Does your digestive system feel heavy?
- Are your bowels moving two to three times a day?
- Do you have great energy levels?
- Do you feel heavy and sluggish?

Ask yourself these questions when it comes to deciding how much meat is the right amount for you and aim to consume only organic and grass-fed sources due to the high amounts of chemicals, antibiotics and hormones livestock are exposed to.

From a spiritual-emotional perspective, also look to source meats that have been ethically farmed. If any animal has undergone stressful living conditions and trauma around the time of slaughter, the emotional stress that is left on the meat will have a significant energetic imprint which will affect your own energy upon consumption.

Meat consumption is a big contributor to colon congestion, infections and liver toxicity as outlined in the previous chapters, so if you do choose to continue to consume, do it responsibly and ensure you undertake multiple colon cleanse protocols each year to maintain the health of your digestive system, microbiome, liver and hormones. If you are open to addressing the ethical and health element of meat consumption there are many great documentaries available such as Forks over Knives, Cowspiracy, Earthlings, What the Health, and Live and Let Live to open your perspective on the consumption of animal products.

Fruit is your friend

Fruit is a classic cyclic symbology of fertility, seeds which sprout, flowers which blossom, bearing fruit providing nourishment for others. Women also possess this same fertile cycle. Fruit is another controversial topic which has created a divide in the nutrition world, with many stuck in fear of the high amounts of natural sugar found in fruit. Yes, fruit has sugar in it, but do you know what your adrenal glands and your brain run off specifically? Sugar, natural sugar. Natural sugar simply cannot harm your body because it always exists symbiotically with the natural fibre, water, antioxidants, vitamins and minerals which balance the overall value of the fruit, preventing dangerous blood sugar spikes or inflammatory effects from the natural sugar. Depriving your body of fruit is a massive disservice which is going to impact your reproductive health, your energy and vitality eventually.

Anti-oxidants are anti-ageing, fruit is high in micronutrients, the healing elements of our food which repair and restore natural balance within the body. Fruit, as it is largely consumed raw which maintains the living enzymes which have the ability to cleanse our blood and lymphatic system, break down cysts, clear out excess mucus and flush the liver. Even with underlying candida conditions, I still do not believe that consuming large amounts of fruit can be a bad thing.

Nutrition for Balanced Hormones

Despite the fact I've been telling you to stop listening to the noise around you and start tuning in, as a nutritionist who specialises in reproductive disorders there are some specific nutritional guidelines that I do believe are paramount to your health journey. And no matter what eating style or diet you choose to follow for you, these are non-negotiables that everyone should be including in their daily considerations with food.

Basic nutritional non-negotiables

- **Meat.** It's not beneficial for everyone. Do your own body investigations.
- **Fruit.** Does not cause candida or cancer. Do your own internal research to feel how it benefits your body.
- **Vegetables.** Eat 10 serves every day.
- **Micros over macros.** Forget about calories, focus on vitamins and minerals.
- **Variety is the spice of life.** Change it up, expose yourself to as many different foods and micronutrients as possible.
- **Consume 50-60% of your food raw daily.** Sounds harder than it is. Snack of raw fruit, nuts and seeds, a cold-pressed juice or smoothie daily, add a salad with lunch or dinner. Done.
- **Beverages are liquid food.** That includes alcohol, coffee and kombucha. Don't forget to consider what you are drinking as part of your daily nutritional intake.
- **Fermented foods aren't for everyone.** Fermented foods are very high in histamines, which can cause problems in some people, particularly those with MTHFR gene mutations and oestrogen dominance. Test and see how it feels for you.
- **Portion size matters.** Overeating, even if it's healthy food will still put a strain on your digestive system, digestive secretions and liver. Eat slowly and allow your brain to process that feeling of fullness before you feel overfull.
- **Don't ever eat something because your coach or nutritionist told you to.** Check in. Does it taste good? Does it feel good? Am I actually hungry?

Step 6 - Nailing Nutrition

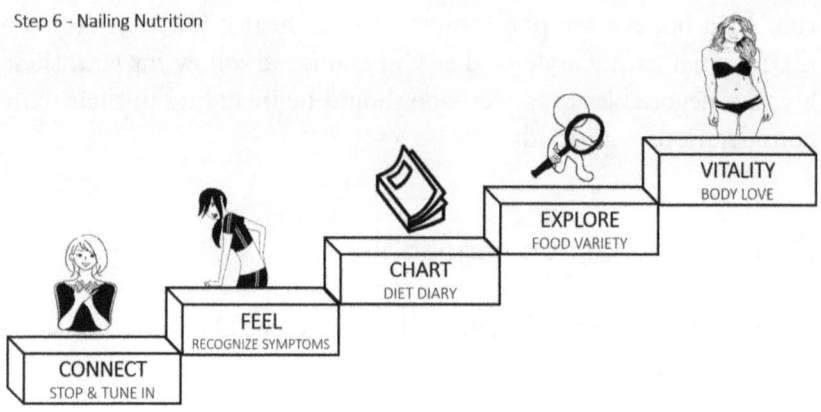

Spiritual shake-up

AWARENESS

Self-awareness gives us the gift of understanding, opening us up to a whole new world of choices, allowing ourselves to experience our best possible life and choose what feels good for us in any given moment. This is an acquired skill which allows us to go within, to listen to our bodies and the messages our hormones are giving us, to feel when our choices and actions are out of alignment and steering us off our path and into discomfort. Having the ability to practice self-awareness in any given situation allows us to foresee future consequences and save ourselves the pain of suffering.

Practising self-awareness is as simple as practising mindfulness in any given moment. To stop and feel before we react and then make decisions based on what feels good for us, rather than what we may believe to be true based upon a preconceived idea or influence of someone else.

Successful self-awareness comes from consistent self-inquiry, which is as easy as asking yourself, how am I feeling, in regards to each situation as it presents. When it comes to understanding food and the effects it has on your body, self-inquiry involves investigating how you physically feel around food and how your current way of eating is affecting you.

Ask yourself:

- Do you have the energy to do all the things that you want to?
- Do you feel energised after eating a meal?
- Do you feel heavy and uncomfortable after eating particular foods?
- Does your concentration wander after certain foods?
- Do you notice your vision changes after certain foods?
- Do you experience skin break-outs after eating certain foods?

After each meal, simply gift yourself the time to be present with your body for just a few moments. This involves stopping whatever you are doing and closing your eyes to shut out external distractions and just feeling. This may only take 30 seconds. The more you can consciously choose to 'check in' like this and in that moment scan your body with awareness and feel how your body is responding post your meal is how you start to build your relationship with food and gain the crucial understanding you need to fuel your body correctly.

ACCEPTANCE

Surrendering to where you are right now is a huge step in taking charge of your body, your health and your relationship with food. When we're caught up in the judgement of how our body looks or why it's not functioning the way we would ideally like it to, we're missing the opportunity to listen to what our body is actually trying to tell us.

- Where are you on your journey right now?
- Do you hate your body, or do you love it?
- Are you confused about what is the right food to eat?
- What emotions or beliefs do you have surrounding your body shape or your physical health?
- Are you an emotional eater?
- Are you a picky eater?
- Do you skip meals and why?

When it comes to healthy whole foods such as fruits and vegetables, get comfortable with exploring your food aversions and delve a little deeper. Why do you hate, for example, brussel sprouts so much? What do they represent to you? Quite often it is much more than just the taste and more so a childhood memory or an association you have with this particular food.

- What are your emotional eating patterns?
- When are you most likely to reach for sugary, salty comfort foods?
- Check in at these times and ask yourself:
    - What is the uncomfortable emotion I am trying not to feel right now?
    - What stories are you running around food?
    - Do you believe cooking is hard or eating healthy food is expensive?

Awareness is the first step and acceptance is the second step. Once we are aware of the stories and issues we have around food, we must then accept this as a crucial part of the journey that must be sat with. This the message your body is trying to give you. The wisdom comes from accepting that this is exactly where you are meant to be right now on your journey and letting go of all judgement around this. Only when we can surrender to the story our ego is telling us and see the beauty in our current situation, are we ready to move forward and make the necessary changes to support our health or change our situation. Accepting the pain and discomfort can be a challenge but until we are willing to change our perception on it and really understand that the body has a bigger purpose than just causing our uncomfortable sensations, we will not be able to change our situation.

ACTION
Implementing change, one day at a time. The final piece of the puzzle is action. Once you have gained the awareness as to what is actually occurring in your body in response to your food and then fully accept that there is a purpose or a reason behind that, then you will be ready to implement the changes to your way of thinking or eating that will help you achieve your health goals.

Creating a food diary

For some this is an extremely tedious process that many resist and if you find the idea of recording what you are eating each day a chore, check in and ask yourself why. What scares you about accountability? In truth, this process really only takes a couple of minutes; simply record everything you ate at the exact time of the day in a journal and then ensure you take the time to implement the mindfulness of checking in and asking yourself how you are feeling. Record all sensations, physical and emotional that you experience each day, using the self-inquiry process to prompt deeper understanding. Each evening when you hop into bed, quickly review your notes and start to take note of any correlations that occur.

Each week set yourself an objection. This could be to identify whether or not meat heals or harms you. So, with the intention experiment with days with meat and days without meat, experiment with meat serving sizes, different types of meat and extended periods without meat and check in regularly until you establish a clear pattern and understanding as to whether or not meat allows you to thrive. Meat is a very broad food group so expect it to take you several months to truly decide whether or not meat is for you or not. Be patient with yourself, be willing to push yourself out of your comfort zone but also don't be hard on yourself if you don't follow through on an intention you have set for yourself on that particular day. Simply ask yourself why you ate something you said you wouldn't and look at the emotions or stories which came up for you. This is a journey. It may take you years to truly understand the exact foods that heal your body and the foods that create inflammation, so enjoy the process and trust that your body has the answers if you are willing to listen.

CHAPTER 11

EMOTIONAL EVOLUTION

"Every man and woman is the architect of their own healing."

Buddha

Hold onto your seats, girlfriend. Things are about to get emotional, but in the best kind of way. Not necessarily an easy topic to talk about, but a very powerful and profound one, especially in terms of connecting with your body and healing your hormones! I truly believe that no disease comes without an emotional trigger. And by that, I mean a trapped or suppressed painful memory that we've not made peace with. Stored emotions that are not expressed freely or simply not heard or felt, become stuck as a dense energy field within our tissues and will eventually lead to stress and dis-ease within the physical body. Generally speaking, pain is the manifestation of trapped emotional trauma that hasn't been resolved, healed and addressed.

A huge part of our healing journey in balancing our hormones, protecting our body, or overcoming a current health hurdle is going to involve identifying the suppressed emotion, most likely from our childhood, which at the time we didn't have the mental and emotional capacity to understand or know how to express safely. So, we found a way to ignore them, distract ourselves from the discomfort or project it onto someone or something else, leaving them buried deep below the surface because it was too painful to experience at the time, or simply finding our way back to our truth and living life in accordance to our highest excitement.

Humans are very clever at avoiding discomfort, especially emotional pain. We've learnt how to ignore anything that doesn't feel particularly good, adopting habits to distract ourselves from the issue at hand. For me it was eating chocolate, when I felt stressed, angry, anxious, sad, depressed or even happiness, which I didn't truly feel worthy of. I would avoid the uncomfortable feeling by over-indulging in chocolate, which gave me something else to fixate on.

Unfortunately, though, over the years we continue to ignore our 'inner child' and the pain we buried with her, and the amount of 'substance' we require to silence the calling continues to increase until the body really screams out for our attention by way of a painful or uncomfortable physical symptom.

When it comes to female reproductive disorders, the womb is a fragile organ due to its nature in 'collecting' and storing dense energy, which is why conditions such as endometriosis, PCOS, pelvic inflammatory disease, sexually transmitted diseases, irregular cervical cells, period pain, fibroids and so forth are such a huge issue affecting one in every five women. The womb space can be likened to a vase, a beautiful, secure container which holds the nourishment for the flowers, keeping them healthy and vibrant, an example of a beautiful, creative, feminine expression of beauty. Our womb and the entire pelvic cavity is a source of nourishment physically and energetically for our entire body and when the energy is flowing freely to that sacred area of our body, like healthy flowers, they open up and bloom. This is exactly the nurturing which the womb provides for our energetic heart space, allowing our heart to open, free to express ourselves creatively, allowing us to give and receive love and follow our hearts' desires.

However, when we are harbouring unexpressed, negative emotions from previous trauma or everyday negative emotions such as shame, guilt, anger, fear, resentment, hate and so forth which are heavy, dense energies, they eventually settle at the bottom of the vase and create stress and tension within that organ, which will eventually manifest as disease. So, when these emotions are not released in a positive manner or transmuted through daily self-care practices, exercise, talking it over with a friend or counsellor, or we simply don't have the tools to gain the awareness of how to heal from these events, eventually our pelvic region will bear the burden.

The truth is, most of us have something we've learnt to implement as a coping mechanism or an avoidance technique to prevent us from feeling uncomfortable emotions. In the short term this is great, it helps us to 'pull on our big girl panties', smile and get on with it. For some women it's retail therapy, the need to be noticed by men, alcoholism, or exercise obsessions. It doesn't particularly matter what the co-dependent activity is, but if you're doing it in an attempt to ignore your intuition or the painful feeling your body is trying to share, you're completely disconnecting from the physical body and silencing your spiritual and emotional connection.

Keeping in mind our hormones are messengers, if we're not listening to what they're trying to tell us about a behaviour or action we're carrying out that is damaging to our physical body, it won't end until we have the awareness. This could be identifying a limiting belief that is stopping us from living the life of our dreams or awareness around a toxic relationship that intuitively we know you need to end but are too afraid to. Our intuition largely uses 'feelings' or emotions to communicate with us. Some of us are lucky enough to hear voices, but for the most part, 'feelings' are our inner compass, designed to direct us away from harm, towards happiness. The only problem is, we're not taught this as children so we're largely a world of zombies walking around completely disconnected from our inner guidance systems, devoid of self-awareness and completely out of touch with the world around us. This not only damages our relationship with ourselves but our friends and family also. If we continue to ignore our 'inner knowing' or 'gut feelings,' we risk becoming more and more out of touch with our higher self and true path and the painful emotions become buried deeper and deeper until they create stress in our organs.

That painful period, cysts on the ovaries, fertility issues and so forth is merely your body trying to communicate with you that there is something below that needs to be addressed, healed and released. Although we have a physical body, we are energetic beings, which is affected by anything and everything in our external environment from the Wi-Fi radiation, to the bad attitude of our work colleague, the toxic foods we put in our body and the negatives belief we carry about ourselves. These all affect our vibration, leading to constriction of the flow of energy through our body, which over time suppresses the immune system, diminishes our vitality and will eventually present itself in the form of disease in our physical body.

Your body is your best friend, communicating with you all the time and constantly trying to protect you and allow you to live your best life. Remembering that symptoms are merely warnings to raise awareness about something which is not functioning smoothly within your body.

Introducing your ego

According to the famous psychologist, Sigmund Freud, the ego is part of the personality that mediates the demands of ID, the superego, and reality. Freud described the ID as the most basic part of the personality that spurs people to fulfil basic primal needs, whereas the super ego works on morals, forming our personality based on the things we were exposed to as children and the values of our immediate upbringing and social influences. It is the ego's job to balance these elements in order to keep life logical, predictable and safe.

I have come to believe that the ego is our friend and although it is a human element which allows us to process the 'reality' of everyday life and make judgements which are necessary for our survival it is also that which creates the illusion of separation. By separation, I refer to the belief that since we inhabit a physical body, we are separate from universal energy, our ego mind identifies us as being separate from the energy but in actual fact energy is everything, be it dense matter or something you can't see, energy is the element which connects us all. The ego also serves to protect us. Without the ability to make judgements based upon our perception of everyday events we would not have the ability to protect ourselves from danger. However, it is this fear of danger which quite often controls our decision making and holds us back from achieving all that we desire.

The ego definitely gets a bad rap. Quite often we're shamed for having a 'big ego', scolded for being egotistical or 'full of ourselves' but essentially your ego is necessary in order to formulate your individual identity and it's not out to ruin your life as you may think. Your ego is required to keep you safe, functioning to keep your reality consistent, predictable and controlled. When your creative mind has a great idea and dares to try something new, it's the ego's job to analyse it, and exhibit caution to prevent you from risking something new which is unfamiliar and therefore dangerous. That's when doubt kicks in and you will find yourself talking yourself out of it, because new is unpredictable and the ego doesn't like that.

The reality is, living life based upon your ego's restraints simply keeps us in the comfort zone and we all know that's not where the magic happens. It happens where we dare to dream, take risks, and flirt with failure. This is largely what being vulnerable is all about, deciding what we want and going for it, even though it's scary and our weaknesses are exposed. This is what having an open heart is all about. It's living life as if nothing else matters, being true to ourselves and our own desires despite the outcomes and the ramifications of how that might look or be perceived by others' judgements. When we can let go of our fear of failure and our fear of judgment, that's when we can truly set ourselves free and that is an untethered soul!

Your thoughts create your reality

As an energetic, vibrating being, we are very much like an antenna, broadcasting our signal based upon the thoughts and emotions we radiate. Good thoughts and feels create a high vibrational frequency which stretches far and wide and is exactly why there are certain people in your world you are subconsciously drawn to and feel great in their company and why you don't feel so excited about life around the negative Nancy's of the world.

Your attitude, thoughts, values and beliefs are the ingredients to the signal you emit, which based on the 'like attracts like' theory will determine the types of people and experience your draw into your reality. If you're walking around feeling like the world's against you, that no one can be trusted and that you always have bad luck, then guess what, these are the things that are going to show up in your reality.

Your external world is always a direct representation of your internal world. And our friends and family will always be our greatest reflections and opportunity for self-evaluation, as they merely act as a mirror to our own soul. If you have 'assholes in your world' why are you attracting them, why are you allowing them in your field and what can you reflect upon their behaviour in terms of how you may be unconsciously carrying out similar behaviour?

Quite often when people are victims of bullying, it's very much a sign that we need to reclaim our personal power. We need to stand up and assert ourselves, not in a reactive kind of way, but more like a, "this is who I am, this is what I stand for, these are my boundaries, and this is what I will and won't tolerate." Boundary setting is about asserting what you will and will not allow others to take from you and is a huge learning experience for many women because it is our natural state to nurture and give to others. Quite often women fall into the trap of giving away their personal power, like expecting someone else to fix us, wanting someone else to rescue us or needing someone else to fill our cup through compliments or acknowledgement, but ultimately, if you aren't your own best friend, if you don't love yourself more than your husband loves you or your children love you, you are setting yourself up for personal heartbreak because you cannot control anyone else's actions or how they treat you except your own.

What is your body trying to tell you about your health?

When it comes to physical illness, I believe you are not at the mercy of some random fate or bad luck and that nothing happens without reason. Classic cause and effect. This can be a particularly hard concept to accept for someone crippled by chronic illness, but as discussed in Chapters 1 and 2, to shift our perception to an opening to see that there is always a blessing in suffering and a lesson to be learnt we are able to take back our personal power.

I believe that everything happens for a reason and for the large part, as a soul choosing to inhabit a human body to experience a human existence, a big part of that is experiencing all emotions, the pleasurable and the not so comfortable. When we can adopt an attitude that everything happens for us, rather than to us, we are able to see everything in our path as an opportunity to grow and learn from, release our judgement and simply let all experiences pass us by and not completely break us.

Spiritual concepts such as these may be a whole new concept to you and for some quite scary, because for a very long time it has been something that science has not been able to measure and therefore classified as 'woo woo'. Our spiritual health is just as important as our physical and emotional health and to ignore this facet of our existence really does shut us off from truly experiencing the magic of creation. When we are able to believe in a power much bigger than ourselves or that which our ego mind would have us believe, we open ourselves up to unlimited possibilities and personal power which allows us to live the life of our dreams, completely supported by the universe and all its energy.

Let's look at PMS, for example. Premenstrual syndrome can manifest as irritability, anger, sadness, sugar cravings, skin breakouts, even physical bloating. But essentially, when you're in that premenstrual phase, that is when our intuition is at its highest and why we feel things more intensely. This is the time to go within, quieten the analytical mind and listen to the signs your body is giving you, physical signs and messages. Why does your partner irritate the crap out of you every month or why do you find yourself in tears dreading going to work before your bleed each month? What is the message? Where are you living out of alignment? This phase of the cycle is when the veil between the conscious and subconscious minds is the thinnest and we are able to hear, feel and see more clearly what our higher self is trying to show us. The premenstrual phase of the cycle is where you will notice the wisdom your body is giving about where you are not living in alignment in accordance to your values, true happiness, where you are living life for someone else on their terms, to make them happy and not valuing your own desires, dreams and passions. In doing so we're essentially disconnected from our soul, which is painful at best, sucking our vitality and diminishing our energetic field, which will show up physically as fatigue, low mood and disease.

Your soul desires to express itself creatively and to do all the things that light you up without fear of others' opinions. When we live in fear, contracted by our own self-judgements and worrying too much about what people think, we are holding ourselves back from our greatest desires and not showing up in our life as our true authentic self, which essentially suffocates our soul.

Your diagnosis doesn't define you, unless you let it. When we become so firmly attached to our diagnosis it becomes our identity and keeps us firmly rooted in the victim state of the disease being completely out of our own control. With a strong sense of your own identity, you are able to create a life that does not include your disease and are able to embody a vibration of someone who is healthy. As Dr Joe Dispenza says, 'The power that made the body, heals the body'. The same lifeforce that has the ability to create life and grow a human being has the ability to heal the body of anything, if we are willing to choose that for ourselves.

Have you ever felt lost, with no reason why? You can't actually explain how you're feeling, but all you know is something doesn't feel quite right. Most people go on to identify this as depression or anxiety, but essentially, this is a feeling of disconnection, when you are living out of alignment. Not speaking your truth, not living your life authentically and not showing up as the person you truly want to be. The problem is a lot of us don't even know who we're supposed to be, what we're supposed to do and how our life is supposed to look, because we're so caught up in the hustle and bustle of everyday life that we don't have a strong understanding of who we are. Our passions, goals, values, desires, needs and wants. When we exist from this shaky foundation with no anchoring to who we truly are, we're more easily influenced by social media, our peers, or even our parents and their values, even if they are not consistent with our own. We become who we think other people want us to be, and live our life based on what we think we should be doing rather than what we choose to be doing. Living out of alignment will always eventually lead to a physical imbalance if you don't course-correct quickly enough.

This scenario commonly plays out in women who have spent their entire motherhood years completely devoted to meeting their children's needs, neglecting their own desires. Then when their children leave home, empty nest syndrome kicks in because they have nothing of their own that brings them joy. Women can plummet into depression and grief, triggering feelings of lack of love and self-worth when they are no longer their children's number one priority, and without a solid foundation of self-love, without their children's constant validation, they feel they have nothing.

Making others' happiness our priority is a dangerous game which at a surface level feels kind and warm to generously give to someone we love. But if we do not know how to balance our energy by giving to ourselves as freely as we give to others, eventually we empty ourselves and have nothing left to give, leaving us feeling depleted, burnt out and resentful. More often than not, that resentment is an unconscious feeling that we are not even aware of because our core belief is that it is our job to make others happy, but this feeling of emptiness and resentment settles heavily within our reproductive organs, including breast tissue, creating stress at a cellular level and eventually disease.

Your purpose

Not everyone is meant to change the world, run charity marathons or make scientific health discoveries. No matter how big or small your mission in life may seem, as long as it excites you and fulfils you, your purpose is what keeps you in alignment with your soul journey. This is what feeling connected to your higher self feels like, feeling joy and excitement every day and feeling like you are following your dreams and making a difference in the lives of those around you. When we are disconnected and don't know who we truly are or have a strong sense of our values, passions and dreams how well do we really know ourselves?

Relationship with yourself - your emotional evolution

You will never evolve if your mind stays in the past, you will simply stay stuck in the same familiar pattern and keep repeating the same familiar mistakes with the same results. A big part of healing our physical body is about having the courage to love yourself enough, to choose yourself and your health above everything else in order to change your circumstances.

Self-esteem has become a big issue which is the core driver of low self-worth and a lack of self-love. How people view us and respond to us is completely out of our control, but the one thing we can take charge of is our relationship and perception of ourselves. Stopping comparing yourself to others is a big part of reigning in your own energy and focusing on you first. A healthy relationship with self is also very much about having a beautiful balance between both masculine and feminine energy, being able to forgive ourselves and respect ourselves enough to walk away from toxic relationships and environments.

Addressing the emotional element of your physical discomfort

Awareness
Understanding and identifying that there is an issue is the first step. Gaining awareness around the situation is about understanding that your physical manifestation is a part of a bigger picture that your body is communicating to you or suffering from the suppressed stress affecting your physical body.

Awareness is gained when we are able to stop, slow down, look, listen and feel into ourselves. This can only be done through a concentrated practice of mindfulness and acknowledging your body on a regular basis. When life is busy, and we're caught up in the 'fast lane' prioritising external things before our own immediate needs and desires, we easily lose touch with what is occurring right under our nose, so to speak.

A great practice for getting back in touch with your body is to ask yourself questions and slow down enough to receive the wisdom your body has to offer through feelings and thoughts which enter your conscious awareness. These answers can even present through things you see, conversations that occur with others or coincidences you start to notices. For example, you may ask your body, what do you need to feel better today and then the first thing you see is an advertisement for an Osteopath. These are not coincidences, rather synchronicities that occur when you open your field and let the universal energy start to communicate with you. Talk to your body and acknowledge it, pay attention to what it is expressing and experiment with different ways of meeting its, your own needs.

Questions to ask include:

- **Where am I not following my heart?**
- **What is the limiting belief that is holding me back?**
- **Where are my everyday actions out of alignment with my values and beliefs?**

The answers will be subtle, especially at first. Learning how to listen to your body is like using a brand new muscle which is small and weak; the only way to strengthen it is to repeatedly practice the action until it becomes more familiar. Journaling is a beautiful way to listen. Ask yourself questions, sit quietly in meditation with your intention in mind, then allow yourself to freely write whatever comes to your head, no matter how irrelevant it may seem. This will always offer guidance if we are willing to listen and see the truth of our ways.

Acceptance

This is where I am right now, and it's okay to feel the way I do. If we are desperately trying to change our circumstances, it's very easy to focus on the future and how we want to feel, but sometimes that in itself misses the messages that our body is trying to share if we cannot be fully present in the moment, right now, and have gratitude for the events that are taking place by seeing the 'blessing' in your suffering we can miss the opportunity to learn. No matter how unfair or painful they may seem, there is always a reason we experience the pain and situations we do and being willing to see these major life interruptions as a course correction helps to keep up moving ahead in the right direction on our true soul path.

Alignment

When we live in alignment with our purpose and our highest joy, our physical health benefits tremendously. Disease cannot exist when our vibration is at its fullest. From a place of alignment, we are able to make the best choices to benefit our physical and emotional health, creating more joy, vitality and abundance in our life. The creation of a perfect life can be achieved by following these three key steps, Awareness, Acceptance and Alignment.

Step 7 - Addressing the Emotional Body of Disease

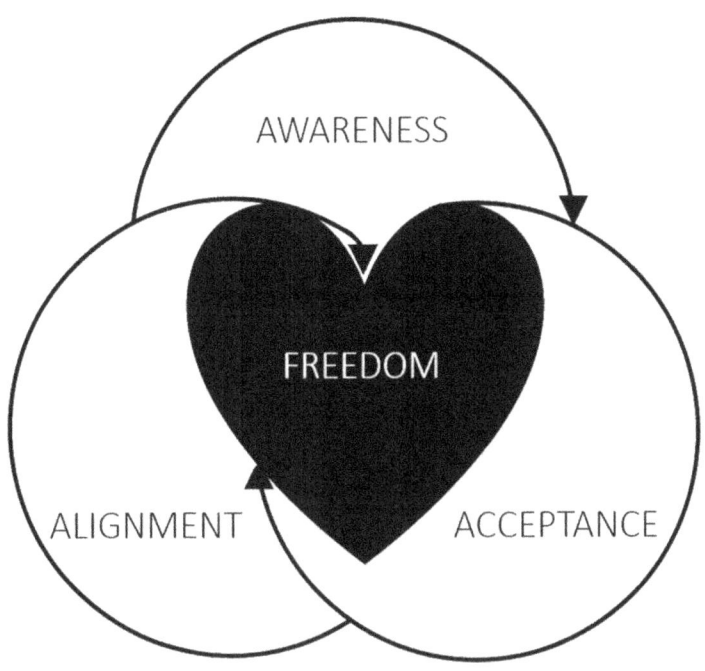

CHAPTER 12

BALANCED & BEAUTIFUL

balance
noun
1.
*An even distribution of weight enabling someone or something to remain upright and steady. "She lost her **balance** and **fell**."*

Life is for living, yeah? I couldn't agree more, in fact, I also tend to think that it's also for testing the limits a little, living large and pushing the boundaries, but the one thing I have learnt both personally and professionally is that 'balance' is the only way to get through life, having lived to the fullest, whilst enjoying the best quality life of all.

I've stressed in this book that I'm a firm believer that the way we live our lives in our earlier years largely defines the quality of our health and experience with life in our later years and if we know better, we can do better.

The average life expectancy in developed countries is increasing and this has improved due to the advancements in medical technology, research in pharmaceuticals, infection control and living standards, however chronic illness disease rate are also significantly increasing, which is severely affecting the quality of human life. We may be living longer, but are we suffering more as a result?

So, where's the balance?

Are we able to live longer and enjoy a higher quality of life, disease and pain-free and stable within our mental, emotional and intellectual health?

For me, balance is about living your best life, experiencing all the fun, adventure, delectable luxuries, pushing ourselves outside of our comfort zones in the pursuit of goal chasing, achievement and accomplishment. We are human after all and we were gifted the seven senses for a reason; Sight, Smell, Taste, Hearing, Touch, Vestibular, Proprioception, all of which allow us to enjoy the world around us and all the beauty it has to offer.

Enjoying life and protecting the human body is about living in balance and respecting our health. It's about understanding how the human body works and what it requires to thrive so that you can make decisions that allow you to enjoy life whilst still supporting your body's needs. Balance is understanding the consequences of your actions and having strategies in place to prevent the aftermath.

The human body is an extremely powerful vessel with no design faults, and when you think about all that we expose our bodies to, the stresses it endures in our lifetimes it's wonderous that we do live as long as we do.

The straw that broke the camel's back

Things such as gluten, heavy metals, fluoride in our water supply, preservatives in our food, which don't have an immediate threat on our health, due to the amazing ability of our body to adapt and protect itself from these carcinogens, will nonetheless have an accumulative effect within the body and eventually cause harm within our major organs.

Worldwide, at least 44 million people are living with dementia, making the disease a global health crisis that must be addressed. (Alzheimer's Association Australia, 2019).

Alzheimer's is a little more difficult to diagnose as the progression of the condition can be slow in onset and misdiagnosed for many years due to the common symptoms of poor memory, problem-solving, task completion and communication, something all of us can relate to from time to time during periods of high stress or fatigue. So, why are our brains becoming so damaged and dysfunctional? Although there are many theories as to why these conditions occur, the cause is still largely unknown according to the medical industry.

As discussed in Chapter 7, dysbiosis is a widespread problem which has a direct impact on the gut-brain axis. Dysbiosis is the overgrowth of pathogenic microbes within the gut flora which is caused by a diet high in gluten, refined sugars and the presence of heavy metals in the absence of beneficial gut flora.

These 'bad' pathogenic gut microbes create increased inflammation systemically and within the gut leading to further problems with obesity, insulin resistance, dysfunctional vago-vagal gut-brain axis. (Daulatzai MA, 2015). And so, we have an indirect correlation between our gut health and brain health which is a widespread cause for the slow long term degeneration of brain function. A problem which if we're made aware of and address through our younger years in life, I believe would have a dramatic improvement in the incidence of these neurodegenerative diseases.[1]

Unfortunately, the 'yolo' approach to life is growing in popularity and due to our overuse and reliance upon something or someone else, being

---

[1] https://www.ncbi.nlm.nih.gov/pubmed/25642988

able to provide 'quick fixes' or lifesaving medical intervention once the 'shit hits the fan' the 'you only live once' reckless approach to self-care is becoming a huge issue later in life, when the damage has been done.

With the emphasis in our current health care system being largely on 'finding cure's' and very little upon prevention, as a society we are becoming people who simply do not know their limits and over-indulge, whether it be risk-taking behaviour, alcohol intake, fast foods or pharmaceutical pill-popping. When we do not have enough self-awareness to consider the long term consequences of our choices, the outcome is more often than not chronic disease that sneaks up on us, all too quickly.

Moving away from this 'all or nothing' mentality is very much about returning to a place of self-respect, listening to our body, learning how to set healthy boundaries and understanding our limits.

Balance - mind - body - soul

Beyond the 7 Step Hormone Healing System, maintaining balance is about creating an environment for you to thrive in and it does require effort. Human health is something that has been taken for granted, as has the treatment of our planet. With pollution levels rising and more and more damage being done to the ozone layer and our environment, human health has become threatened. No longer is 'good health' our divine right, it is something we must claim for ourselves by choosing to live life in a supportive manner to protect the body from the rising amounts of toxicity in our world.

Mental-emotional balance

Protect your energy
Energy vampires are emotionally immature with an inability to see things from other peoples' perspective, believing the whole world revolves around them. Quite often you feel exhausted as if you've had

the life sucked out of you after spending time with these sort of people. It can be very stressful when close friends or family members in your life drain your energy like this. Learning how to protect your energy is an important skill which involves having the capacity to self-reflect and set boundaries. When we are aware of energy-sucking behaviour it is easier to put measures in place which limit our time with these people or adopt methods to dissociate from the behaviour and not take their views and needy behaviour on board, as well as preventing you from compromising your own ethics, values and morals.

Social media
Social media can very much be a positive or negative influence in your life, depending on your own core foundation of self-worth and knowing of who you are. When we are feeling low it is very easy to compare ourselves to others, which is unrealistic when viewing peoples' lives through 'rose coloured' social media glasses and filters. Check in before you aimlessly scroll through social media platforms. How are you feeling and what is your aim for participating in social media? If you are not feeling great about yourself, looking to social media for a quick dopamine hit is a sure-fire way to dig yourself into a deeper hole. Having a strong connection with who you are and the things which bring joy into your life is a great way to fill your own cup without seeking external validation. Make a list of all the things you can think of which make you happy; these can be people, places, things you do, hobbies and so forth. The idea is to create a list of at least 50 things and store it somewhere handy you have easy access to, like the notes section of your phone. Every time you are feeling low you can connect with your list and feel your energy start to improve simply by switching your focus and choosing an activity which will make you feel good in the moment.

Meditation
There are many ways to meditate and whether or not you choose a formal practice, learning how to quieten the mind, go within and silence the outside world is a great way to rejuvenate your mental and emotional health. Meditating for just five minutes a day can provide a significant improvement in your ability to remain calm in stressful

situations and relax the body and the mind and is a great way to practice more self-awareness.

Challenge your brain
Use it or lose it! The more we use our brain, the more we strengthen neural pathways, and we even have the ability to form new neural pathways, improve brain neuroplasticity and strengthen brain cell connections. It's great to stretch your mental capacity by challenging yourself with new tasks which stimulate brain activity, such as reading, learning new skills, learning a foreign language, researching topics you enjoy or participating in crossword puzzles and sudoku.

Physical balance

Body movement and exercise
Movement keeps us flexible, alive and energised. Find a way to enjoy moving your body every single day. There are so many options for this vital process which supports our immune system, improves circulation and boosts mood, so choose something fun that you know you can commit to, even if it's a 5-minute dance around the house each morning. Something is better than nothing, although aiming for 20 minutes five times a week is a great goal. Swim, walk, play, dance, jump, lift, cycle, skate, stretch - the options are unlimited!

Airflow
Ensuring your sleeping environment is well-ventilated is crucial for lung health and general wellbeing. If your climate doesn't permit sleeping with a window open it's a great idea to at least have a fan in your room to keep the air circulating. Sleeping in air-conditioned rooms can lead to irritation of mucus membranes, which can lead to breathing difficulties as well as dry skin and the increased risk of stagnating airflow, allowing germs and micro-organism to breed in the environment. If you work in an office, at the very least make an effort to spend your lunch break outdoors and schedule time outdoors in nature as often as you can.

Immune Support

If there's something you choose to actively supplement your lifestyle with, practices which strengthen and build the production of white blood cells is a major consideration. Viral infections are noted as being something that once we have been exposed to will remain in our systems forever, wreaking havoc behind the scenes and disarming our immune system, linking their involvement with auto-immune conditions and cancer. Supplementing with anti-viral herbs and nutrients to focus on:

- Zinc
- Vitamin C
- Lysine
- Garlic
- Echinacea
- Elderberry
- Astragalus
- Cat's claw
- Reishi, shiitake, turkey tail, lion's mane and Chaga mushrooms
- Olive leaf
- Red clover
- Siberian ginseng

These are all great safe, long-term immune-supporting natural plants or vitamins/miners to build immunity and fight infections. If you are a tea drinker, *purchasing loose leaf herbs is a cost-effective way to consume these herbs.*

Immune-boosting foods:
- Garlic
- Green tea
- Shitake mushrooms
- Sweet potato
- Kale
- Carrots
- Brazil nuts
- Spinach
- Almonds
- Avocado

These foods all have great immune-boosting properties which are great to include in your diet on a regular basis. You cannot overdose on mother nature's gifts, foods which are whole and require no processing for consumption. The more you are able to incorporate these foods daily, the more your body will thrive.

Superfoods

Superfoods are mother nature's gifts. They have high amounts of naturally occurring antioxidants, nutrients and minerals and should be consumed as often as possible to boost your nutritional intake, immune system and support overall health.

Almonds	**Cabbage**	**Goji Berries**	**Pepitas**
Acai berry	**Cacao**	**Green Tea**	**Pineapple**
Apricots	**Carrot**	**Hemp seeds**	**Pomegranate**
Apples	**Cauliflower**	**Kale**	**Potato**
Artichokes	**Chia seeds**	**Kiwi fruit**	**Radish**
Asparagus	**Cherries**	**Lemons & Limes**	**Rocket**
Avocado	**Coconut**	**Lentils**	**Quinoa**
Banana	**Coriander**	**Mangoes**	**Sesame seeds**
Basil	**Cauliflower**	**Microgreens**	**Spinach**
Beans	**Chia seeds**	**Mushrooms**	**Sprouts**
Beetroot	**Dulse**	**Oranges**	**Sweet potato**
Berries	**Grapes**	**Oregano**	**Sunflower seeds**
Broccoli	**Garlic**	**Papaya**	**Tomatoes**
Brussel sprouts	**Ginger**	**Peaches**	**Walnuts**

Regular cleansing

Commit to cleansing your colon several times a year, especially if you choose to consume animal proteins. It's also a great idea to do a liver cleanse protocol at least once a year. Heavy metal detoxing is something that may also need considering; we are all exposed to an alarmingly high amount of heavy metals especially aluminium, cadmium, mercury, lead and arsenic, especially in our water supply, pharmaceutical agents, environmental chemicals and the soil. A heavy metal detoxification program should only be done under the care and close observation of a qualified practitioner but is definitely something that is indicated in chronic health conditions such as auto-immune disorders and inflammation.

Enemas are a personal care practice which I highly recommend should be done several times a week, or as often as you can make time for at the very least.

Check out the Balanced Babes website for specific colon cleansing and liver cleansing protocols and eating plans. https://balancedbabes.net/enemas

Home detoxification

To ensure your hormones remain balanced and your body has the best chance of avoiding chronic disease, it's important that your living environment is a safe, supportive environment for your cells to thrive in. This involves eliminating toxic cleaning chemicals and replacing these with safer, 'greener' brands. Absorbing and counteracting radiation from sources such as the microwave, mobile phones, modems and other smart appliances in the home is paramount. There have been multiple studies done over time which have concluded that the accumulation effect and consistent exposure to these things increase the risk of spontaneous abortion, increased childhood cancers, shifts in white and red blood cell counts and increased somatic mutation in lymphocytes. There's no doubt that these mod cons are highly convenient, and balance is not about throwing every modern-day luxury in the bin but putting steps in place to protect from the damage. A popular, cost-effective step to reducing radiation exposure is to place shungite throughout your home and office. This is a naturally-occurring crystal made of 90% carbon which protects from electro-magnetic radiation and particularly the latest radiation from 5G technology.

Additionally, having indoor plants inside your home is a great way to support health and disease prevention. NASA scientists are finding them to be surprisingly useful in absorbing potentially harmful gases and cleaning the air inside homes, indoor public spaces and office buildings. Sick building syndrome is becoming a well-known issue due to the increasing amounts of gases and indoor pollutants in the home and workplace. Formaldehyde, volatile organic compounds (benzene and trichloroethylene or TCE), airborne biological pollutants, carbon monoxide and nitrogen oxides, pesticides and disinfectants (phenols), and radon have been identified to be the worst culprits but in a two-year study conducted by NASA, over 50 indoor plants were found to be effective in protecting and removing the harmful toxins with the following being the most common and easy to access:

- Areca Palm (Chrysalidocarpus lutescens)
- Lady Palm (Rhapis excelsa)
- Bamboo palm (Chamaedorea seifrizii)
- Rubber Plant (Ficus robusta)
- Dracaena (Dracaena deremensis)
- Philodendron (Philodendron sp.)
- Dwarf Date Palm (Phoenix roebelenii)
- Ficus Alii (Ficus macleilandii "Alii")
- Boston Fern (Nephrolepis exaltata "Bostoniensis")
- Peace Lily (Spathiphyllum "Mauna Loa")

Meal Preparation

When it comes to cooking and meal prep, the first thing you want to do is turf your microwave or at the very least restrict it to emergency use only. Cooking with a microwave oven is highly convenient - it's simple and incredibly fast - however, there has been a lot of debate surrounding the immediate effect it has on the quality of our food and the long-term safety effects.

Microwaves produce electromagnetic waves which stimulate the water molecules in food causing them to vibrate, spin and clash with each other, in turn converting the energy into heat. Although the radiation which is produced is quite low compared to a mobile phone for example, due to the changes it produces on the water molecules within food, particularly fruits and vegetables, plants lose the electromagnetic spark that delivers vital life force to your body's cells; that same energy catalyses beneficial changes within our cells regarding intracellular communication. The truth is, any form of heating food, be it steaming, boiling, baking or frying reduces the nutrient levels in our food and microwaves are no better or worse, but the fact that microwaving leads to the isomerisation of amino acids within proteins is concerning. This is the process by which the amino acid form is converted to a D-form from an L-form, which can't be efficiently digested by humans. Try to consume a diet of up to 70% raw food each day, which is largely possible through the ingestion of cold-pressed juicing, smoothies, salads, fruit, vegetables, nuts, seeds and raw desserts, this is the best way to ensure you are receiving adequate enzymes and nutrition in your diet.

Feminine care
For sanitary items for menstruating women, moving away from tampons can make a huge difference to period pain. Within the United States and many other countries there are no mandatory guidelines for the materials used in feminine hygiene products, which means manufacturers are not required to disclose the ingredients, including chemicals used in the manufacturing process. Tampons are typically made from rayon, viscous and wood fluff pulp, all forms of wood cellulose which is largely treated with dioxin, which is derived from the same family as Agent Orange and is a by-product of pollution from incinerators, pesticide spraying, and the production of paper and rayon products, such as tampons, coffee filters, toilet paper, and even disposable diapers.

According to studies, dioxin can accumulate in the fatty tissues of animals and humans, where it can cause immune system suppression, abnormal tissue growth in your abdomen and reproductive organs, abnormal cell growth throughout your body and hormonal and endocrine system disruption. According to the US Environmental Protection Agency (EPA), dioxin is a serious public health threat and there is no safe level of exposure. To complete the polished appearance of tampons, they are bleached with chlorine to give the appearance of purity and cleanliness, another chemical our sensitive vaginal tissue is exposed to through the use of tampons. Even if you are purchasing organic tampons, although better, the harsh fibres within tampons are very abrasive to the fragile cells of the vaginal wall, creating tiny micro-tears which cause inflammation and an increased risk of bacterial overgrowth in the warm, moist region of the vaginal canal.

I highly recommend the use of permanent personal hygiene products such as period knickers, reusable bamboo cloth pads and reusable menstrual cups which are not only safer for your body but also kinder on the environment and landfill. There will always be occasions when it is more convenient to use a tampon, but in these cases always choose an organic brand and limit your use and don't make it a regular thing.

Beauty Care Products
The other key practice to implement is cleaning up your beauty regime. With so many unregulated toxins circulating in the industry and so many products being applied to female hair, skin and nails daily, it's no wonder our hormones are struggling to do their job effectively, railroaded by endocrine-disrupting molecules which interfere with our normal hormone signalling.

Nowadays there are many chemical-free natural and mineral-based beauty products which are becoming more and more affordable and a fast-growing and competitive industry, so make this one a priority to implement as soon as possible. At the very least, please start by throwing out your aluminium-based deodorant.

Household Appliances
Through my years of research and use, there are several items I have found to be worthwhile investments that I believe every home should

make a priority to repair damage to our cells through everyday living. Here is the list of the top health investments that are worth researching and budgeting for:

- **Home water filtration and ioniser** (even if you use rainwater)
- **Cold-pressed juicer**
- **Good quality blender or food processor**
- **Infrared sauna**
- **Essential oil diffuser** - multiple for bedrooms is a great idea
- **Dehumidifier/Air purifier** for the prevention of mould growth
- **Natural wax or beeswax food covers**, which can be used in the place of plastic food wrap
- **Glass storage containers** (rather than plastic)
- **Enema Kit**

Check out the resources page at https://balacedbabes.net/resources/ for full details of recommended brands of all of the above changes to implement.

Spiritual balance

Self-Awareness
I have touched on self-awareness multiple times in this book. It really is about learning how to take the steering wheel of your own ride and learning how to respond to your ever-changing environment that comes along with life. With good self-awareness it's much easier to 'know your limits' and create better accountability for yourself. So, check in constantly - how are you feeling about the situation? And most importantly, give yourself permission to feel good. Seek support, ask for help and be assertive of your worthiness. You are allowed to have great things in your life, just don't be an asshole in the process.

Self-Care
Self-care should be a hobby, not a chore, and if you're avoiding it because you think you can't be bothered, then you're doing it wrong!

Self-care is especially self-love in motion, it's the acts of kindness to appreciate yourself, nurture yourself and start to reconnect with your body so you can feel what is actually going on for you. It's very much about stopping and taking time out from your mundane daily tasks and making time for things which help you to feel better. This can be as simple as taking a bath, booking yourself in for a massage, seeing your Osteopath or getting your hair done. It can be taking that yoga class or scheduling a date night just for you, time out away from responsibility to be present with yourself and meet your own needs. Self-care is fun if you are doing it right and the only way to do it right is to find the things that leave you feeling great as a result; the calming, relaxing, restorative soul-reviving processes which force you to focus on you, let go all the other identities you are carrying around and get really real with yourself. It's about taking off the mask and showing up in your true essence, free to be you! It's ok to give to you first!

Self-Creation
Owning your thoughts and understanding that you create your reality is a powerful way to improve the level of positivity in your life, be it at home, work or within relationships. Adopting a 'glass half full' approach to life and learning to laugh at yourself more and look on the bright side is a great way to keep your vibration lifted and attract more of those feel-good vibes in the world around you.

Self-Exploration
This is a simple process of getting to know your true self, deep below the superficial layers and identifying your core values, beliefs and true passions. Ask yourself:

- Who am I?
- What am I passionate about?
- What do I stand for?
- What is my purpose?

Humans are naturally creative beings and expressing creatively allows us to live in our truth and discover who we are. When we are disconnected from creative outlets, whether that be drawing, painting, singing, dancing, speaking, writing or any form of personal expression, we become contracted and withdrawn, which drains our physical energy.

There are always going to be situations in your life where it is unrealistic and impractical to completely avoid exposure to harmful things, especially when it comes to fun and recreation, convenience and indulging in guilty pleasures. I for one love my sweets, which is why I've made balance such a huge part of my lifestyle and am able to maintain healthy, happy, balanced hormones, my ideal body weight, healthy skin and mood in spite of probably consuming refined sugar too much.

Whether or not you believe in life after death, we really do get just one chance at life and it's crazy how fast the years pass us by. They say the one regret of the dying is the things they never tried, being ignorant to self-love and self-care which resulted in shorter life spans, and not believing in themselves enough to follow through.

You are a beautiful, powerful creative being with unlimited opportunity to create the life of your dreams when you are willing to get out of your limiting 'stories' and beliefs, so please take this book and go and live an empowered life!

I hope that the information provided in this book has helped you gain an understanding of how and why it is so important to listen to the cues your body is giving you and intervene before chronic illness sets in and you can enjoy the experimenting and self-discovery along the way.

Stay connected

If you want to stay in the loop with women's health and hormone issues and connect with like-minded babes on your journey, please check out our free online community on Facebook Balanced Babes.

Join the Balanced Babes Facebook Group https://www.facebook.com/groups/balancedbabes4life

AFTERWORD

The Balanced Babes Mission

I have a vision and it involves the end of suffering for all women. No more chronic period pain, debilitating PMS, internal struggling, unnecessary removal of uteruses, distressing surgeries and most importantly no more breast cancers.

To empower and educate women with the knowledge of self-awareness, teaching them how to connect with their physical body and learning how to understand why their hormones are 'behaving badly'.

I believe a world without breast cancer is possible, but I need your help. Driving down breast cancer incidence starts with you! Making your health a priority and loving your body enough to take care of it.

Divine woman, your body is a beautiful miracle and when fully connected with your feminine power you are unstoppable!

So, where to from here?

Chronic illness does not have to be part of your journey, if we choose to love, honour and listen to our body and take a proactive stance on 'disease prevention'.

With an understanding that our hormones are merely messengers, relaying the information of a much bigger issue, we are able to take back our power, jump into the driver's seat of our individual health journey, leaving behind feelings of helplessness, being misunderstood and completely overwhelmed by the enormity of our physical health.

If the message and information in this book resonates and you too would like to see an end in chronic illness, I would love for you to help by sharing this book with all the women in your world. From teenage girls to reproducing ladies and even peri- and post-menopausal women, it's never too early or too late to start your empowered health journey and learn how to listen to your hormones.

Together, we can make a difference.

Here's to health & happiness

Stacey Xx

ABOUT THE AUTHOR

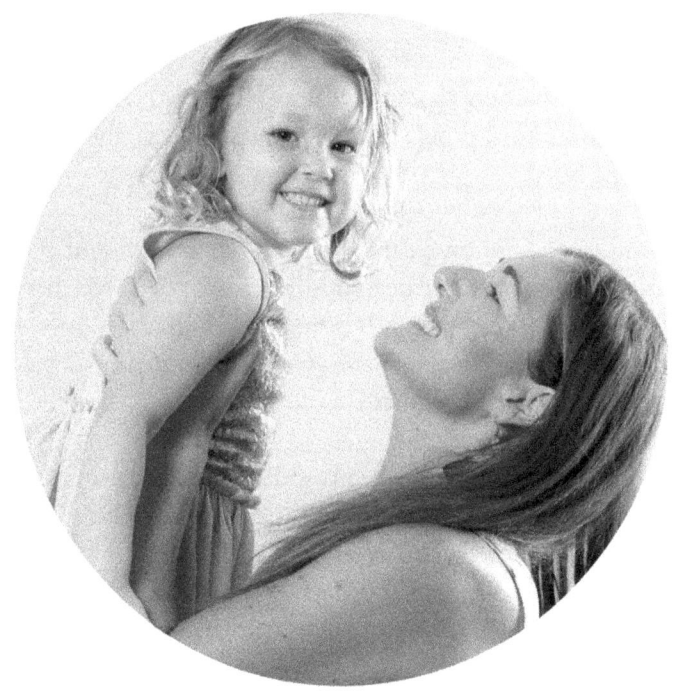

Stacey graduated from the Australian College of Natural Medicine in 2007 with a Bachelor of Health Science, a degree in Nutritional Medicine, an Advanced Diploma of Naturopathy and Certificate IV in Massage.

As the mother of a happy, healthy daughter, Stacey is passionate about allowing women the right and choice to bear children and feel completely at ease and in control of their bodies by understanding how to listen to their hormones, knowing their choices and feeling confident enough to choose the right options for themselves in all elements of women's hormone and reproductive health.

Through her own personal battle with troubled periods, polycystic ovarian syndrome, premature ovarian failure and adrenal fatigue, Stacey seeks to bridge the gap between conventional medicine and natural holistic therapies by empowering and educating women to take a stand for their health and making disease-preventing a priority through making positive lifestyle choices while still enjoying the finer things in life.

This is what inspired the creation of 'Balanced Babes', an online community for women to connect and feel heard, as well as online educational programs, group healings, natural medicine supplements and now this book.

Having suffered for many years with low self-esteem and poor body image, Stacey's journey has been a rollercoaster of yo-yo dieting and 'quick fix' pill-popping, which has taught her that the only real 'fix' is listening to your body and understanding the messages it is trying to give you through discomfort.

"I suffered from severe eczema in my childhood and most of my adult life, until age 30. I wasn't tuning in and aware of the foods which supported my system, I was merely giving away my power, following social media and copying what others were doing in the elusive quest to 'lose weight'. When I learnt to slow down and take notice of the changes occurring in my body, I was able to determine what foods healed and what foods harmed, and I've never had eczema since."

Stacey continues to expand her knowledge through ongoing education and training in modalities such as The Emotional Freedom Technique (EFT), Timeline Therapy, Body Consciousness Therapy, Reiki and is currently undertaking a Womb Awakening Apprenticeship through the Institute of Feminine Arts. She believes physical health is not just a result of our lifestyle choices or genetics, but also largely influenced by our emotional wellbeing, thoughts and neural programming.

Stacey's mission is to dramatically reduce chronic illness such as endometriosis, fibromyalgia, MS and breast cancer, and common female health problems, by empowering and educating women to wellness, reconnecting them with their intuition, enabling them to love and accept themselves and care for their bodies from a place of inner wisdom, full knowing and unwavering self-respect.

ACKNOWLEDGEMENTS

TESTIMONIAL

Nikki, 38, Sunshine Coast, Australia

High school was hard enough without the added pressure of painful, heavy periods. I struggled every month from the age of 13 with mood swings and long, heavy periods that usually left me with period pain for three weeks out of four. Most doctors had brushed me off over the years and told me it was normal to have period pain and experience mood swings. I was prescribed the contraceptive pill and told that I would always have to be on it to balance my period.

Then at the age of 24, I was diagnosed with severe endometriosis. I had surgery to remove the legions that had grown throughout my abdomen and had a Mirena inserted to cease my cycle so the endometriosis would not come back too quickly. They advised I should think about having babies right away as I may have trouble conceiving later in life as the endo would continue to get worse. Four years later, the Mirena moved inside my uterus and I had to have it removed immediately. At 29 years old, I fell pregnant after 12 months of trying.

A couple of years after the birth of my daughter I was back on the operating table to have the endo removed and another Mirena inserted.

I had that Mirena for five years when it began failing and I had massive breakthrough bleeding for two to three weeks per month. My doctor removed the Mirena and put me on a drug to lessen the flow of my period and another one to reduce my period pain. I took these for several months but was not having very good results, so I went back and was told at the age of 37 years that I should strongly consider having a full hysterectomy as there weren't any other options. I declined having a hysterectomy and they put me on progestogen tablets to match my elevated levels of oestrogen (reasons why were not actually explained to me).

Within four months I began having pregnancy symptoms coupled with hot flushes, not to mention the heavy, long painful periods. It was at this point I knew I needed to find an alternative to what the mainstream medical system was offering. This was exactly when Stacey entered my life. Within just a few months of following the advice she gave and taking the supplements she advised based on her 7 Step Hormone Healing System, I was mostly pain-free each month, I didn't experience heavy periods and I didn't have any mood swings. I am so very grateful for the help so far and will continue to work with Stacey until I have a completely normal cycle, something I now see is possible. Stacey has achieved more through a natural alternative in a few months than doctors in the medical world were able to do in 15 years.

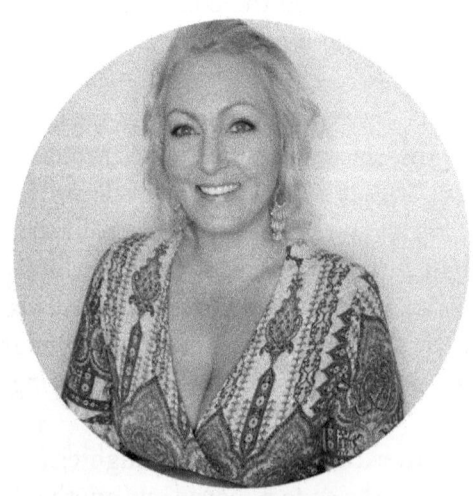

STACEY A FOAT

BALANCED BABES

Founder of Balanced Babes
Author · Speaker · Hormone Specialist

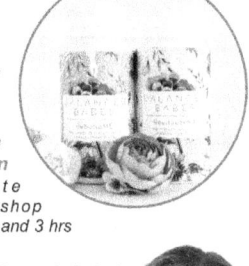

As a qualified Naturopath & Nutritionist Stacey is passionate about teaching women the art of listening to their bodies to understand their hormones. Suffering from Poly cystic ovarian syndrome, many years of debilitating periods and eventually being told she had commenced Menopause at age 27 and would never conceive naturally, Stacey has overcome her own 'hormone hell' and is committed to helping other women heal from the same debilitating diagnosis. Stacey is the proud mother of a beautiful naturally conceived daughter and is determined to bridge the gap between Modern medicine and holistic health by empowering women to make informed decisions about their health and the ability to recognize when something is out of balance before disease sets in. Her ultimate mission is to put an end to debilitating chronic diseases such as Endometriosis, Auto-immunity, Breast and Cervical cancers by teaching women how to care for their bodies.

Balanced Babes

Empowering & Educating Women to Wellness
Connecting women with their hormones & inspiring them to take a stand for their bodies by changing the face of Self Care to a place of self-love and self-respect.

Womb Awakening Guiding women back to their innate wisdom and reconnecting with their intuition.

Hormone Balancing & Cleansing Facilitating the natural healing process of the body by addressing the cause of hormonal imbalances through nutrition correction, detoxification & healing emotional traumas.

Signature Services:

Balance Me™ Online Health Program for Women

The 7 Step Hormone Healing System utilized to heal conditions such as Endometriosis, PCOS, Auto-Immunity, Infertility and prevention of Reproductive and Breast cancer.

The Balanced Babes Sisterhood™

Uniting women and sharing the self-discovery and healing journey with woman wanting to take ownership of their bodies and lives. Online hangouts, and connection circles and healing retreats for birth trauma releasing.

Balanced Babes Professional Health Supplements

Herbal, Nutritional and functional food formulas to restore balance and facilitate holistic healing and hormone balance.

'A passionate and knowledgeable speaker who engages her audiences from the start, Stacey can deliver a key-note presentation or workshop ranging between 45 mins and 3 hrs on the following...

'Hormone Hell to Balanced Babe'
Learning the language of your body, listening to your hormones & stepping into your empowered best self.

'End your Endo' Using holistic therapies to eliminate Endometriosis.

'The Pill Pandemic'
Raising awareness surrounding the dangers of the OCP, how to maintain your natural hormonal rhythm and natural alternatives to synthetic hormones.

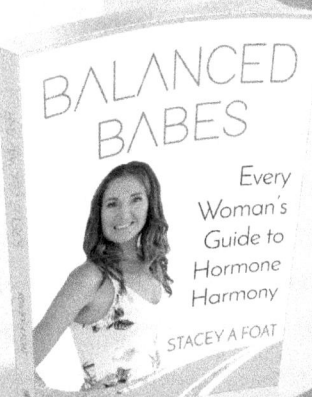

✉ stacey@balancedbabes.net
🖳 www.staceyfoat.com
🖳 www.balancedbabes.com.au

For enquiries please contact Stacey 📱 +61 418 134 883

BALANCED BABES

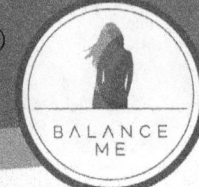

Balance Me - The 7 Step Hormone Healing Program

"Hormone hell to Balanced Babe"

An online, holistic hormone healing program designed to guide women through the 7 Step Hormone Healing system with additional support & mentoring.

In this interactive, educational program you'll address the physical, emotional & spiritual elements of your health by tackling the source of your hormone imbalance to transform your body from 'Hormonal Hell to Balanced Babe'.

What causes Hormone Imbalances?

Toxicity, Nutritional Depletion, Chronic Infection, Immune dysfunction, Stress & living out of alignment, disconnected from your truth!

Hormone Hell To Balanced Babes

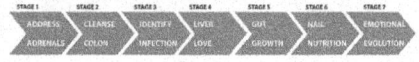

Who is this program for?

Women of all ages who are experiencing any of the following:
- Painful monthly periods
- Hormonal acne
- Fertility problems
- Cysts or fibroids
- Adrenal fatigue
- Thyroid dysfunction
- Hot flushes and debilitating Menopause
- Hormonal mood swings, anxiety or depression
- Loss of libido
- Weight gain

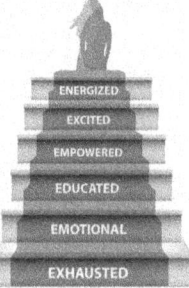

Balance Me TM – Program Includes

- **8 x Naturopathically designed Balanced Babes Hormone Healing Supplements**

- **Balanced Babes Sisterhood Access**
  Online group healing sessions to address limiting beliefs & facilitate emotional evolution

- **The Balance Me Online Education Program**
  12 core modules including videos, downloads & checklists

- **Eating Plans**
  3 different stages with shopping lists, menu planner & recipes

- **DIY Treatment Protocols**
  Specific instructions for treating all common 'symptoms' associated with Hormonal imbalances from candida infections, migraines, hormonal acne and more!

- **12 x weekly ACTION Plans**
  Including: Castor oil packing, Enema's, Cleansing & signature Balanced Babes Hormone Healing practices

- **Downloadable PDFs**
  Includes checklists, guides, instructions, recipes

- **Weekly Accountability Emails to keep you motivated**

- **Referral for General & Functional Pathology**
  With detailed analysis & recommendations for results

- **VIP Balanced Babes exclusive Membership Group**
  Share the journey with other women for additional support

Book a **FREE 30 minute** Hormone Assessment to help kick start your transformation.
http://bit.ly/hormoneassessment

Your ideal body, healthy skin, endless energy & healthy libido is just some of the benefits of the Balance Me Program
For further enquires: stacey@balancedbabes.com.au
www.balancedbabes.com.au

www.ingramcontent.com/pod-product-compliance
Lightning Source LLC
Chambersburg PA
CBHW031150020426
42333CB00013B/595